INTRODUCTION TO RADIOLOGY IN CLINICAL PEDIATRICS

INTRODUCTION TO RADIOLOGY IN CLINICAL PEDIATRICS

JACK O. HALLER, M.D.

Professor of Clinical Radiology
State University of New York
Downstate Medical Center
Director of Pediatric Imaging
Kings County Hospital Center
Brooklyn, New York

THOMAS L. SLOVIS, M.D.

Clinical Associate Professor of Radiology
Associate in Pediatrics
Wayne State University School of Medicine
Radiologist
Children's Hospital of Michigan
Detroit, Michigan

With the assistance of
JOSEPH O. REED, M.D.,
Professor of Radiology, Director of Radiology,
Children's Hospital of Michigan,
Detroit, Michigan

YEAR BOOK MEDICAL PUBLISHERS, INC.

CHICAGO • LONDON

Library of Congress Cataloging in Publication Data

Haller, Jack O.
   Introduction to radiology in clinical pediatrics.

   Includes index.
   1. Pediatric radiology.   I. Slovis, Thomas L.
II. Title. [DNLM: 1. Radiography—In infancy and child-
hood. WN 240 H185i]
RJ51.R3H34   1983   618.92′007572   83-5878
ISBN 0-8151-4108-4

To ADOLF *and* FRIEDA HALLER,
my mentors, my inspiration, my parents.

J.O.H.

To ELLIE, MICHAEL, DEBBIE, ANDY, *and* LISA,
my family, without whose love, patience, and inspiration
this project could not have been completed.

T.L.S.

Contents

Preface

THE IDEA for this book grew out of our experiences in teaching pediatric radiology to clinicians and students. Clearly, there is a strong desire on the part of those taking care of children to familiarize themselves with the rudiments of the pediatric radiograph. While radiologists have primary responsibility for the interpretation of films, clinicians bring valuable insight and information. Often they present additional important data or ask searching questions that prompt a re-evaluation of the films so that a more appropriate diagnosis may be obtained.

While primers are available in adult radiology, comparable editions in pediatrics are lacking. We have therefore adapted the teaching sessions of Joseph O. Reed, Director of Radiology at Children's Hospital of Michigan, and Professor of Radiology at Wayne State University School of Medicine, as the framework for our text. In addition, Rosalind H. Troupin* has generously allowed us to use some of her ideas for this book, which is an elementary guide to common pediatic radiographic examinations and problems. It is our intent to provide an approach to these examinations to help the clinician discern the normal from the abnormal. A second goal is to help the pediatrician, house officer, and medical student learn the indications for various procedures, as well as to recognize some of the more common abnormalities. This text is by no means meant to provide an in-depth discussion of various disease entities, nor is it intended to catalog the various subtle radiographic findings in these entities.

The radiographs in this volume are often reproduced to enhance a single finding under discussion, often at the expense of other portions of the film. Also, arrows and letters have been kept to a minimum so as not to obscure the radiographs.

It is our hope that, by providing this primer for pediatric radiology, we will stimulate clinicians to visit the x-ray department, share in the interpretation of their patients' films, and continue to stimulate us so that together we can provide optimal care for children.

JACK O. HALLER

THOMAS L. SLOVIS

---

*Troupin R. H.: *Diagnostic Radiology in Clinical Medicine*, ed. 2. Chicago: Year Book Medical Publishers, Inc., 1978.

Acknowledgments

WE WISH TO ACKNOWLEDGE a number of individuals without whom this work would not have been completed. Drs. Ronald L. Poland, John K. Kelly, Harvey I. Wilner, and Alfredo Lazo offered helpful criticisms of early drafts. Drs. Alkis Zingas, Alfredo Lazo, and Lawrence R. Kuhns were kind enough to lend us computerized tomographic images and the nuclear medicine images found within the text. Virginia Newman did yeoman work in typing and retyping numerous revisions of this manuscript over a two-year period. Without her hard work, the task would have been impossible.

Albert Paglialunga and Shelley Eshelman provided the reproductions of the radiographs and the schematic diagrams, respectively. They were patient and responsive.

Dr. Joshua A. Becker, a chairman and friend, has continued to provide support and encouragement for academic pursuits and sustains a gratifying working milieu.

Drs. George B. Comerci, Lewis A. Barness, and C. Henry Kempe stimulated our interest in pediatrics and urged close rapport with our pediatric colleagues. Dr. R. Parker Allen has been responsible for first "turning on" many of his students to radiology.

Drs. David H. Baker and Walter E. Berdon, our mentors, godfathers, and friends, have always encouraged us and continue to serve as models of excellence in pediatric radiology.

Dr. Joseph O. Reed (whose Reed's Rules appear throughout this book), has helped with his guidance, teaching, and critical appraisal of the manuscript. He has provided this stimulus by emphasizing basic principles as a means to learning radiology and, in fact, medicine itself.

CHAPTER 1

Radiographs and Their Use

NATURE OF RADIOGRAPHS

X-RAYS are short electromagnetic radiations "produced by energy conversion when fast-moving electrons from the filament of the x-ray tube interact with the tungsten anode (target)"[1] (Fig 1–1). When an x-ray beam is directed toward a part of the body, x-rays are absorbed by the more dense tissue (e.g., bone). X-rays that pass through the entire body interact with the x-ray film (intensifying screens, etc.), forming an image, while absorbed x-rays cause ionization within the body. The x-ray picture, or radiograph, is a recording of internal body structures where the black areas represent regions that have allowed the x-rays to pass through and onto the film and the white areas the regions that have absorbed all x-rays before they reach the film. Thus, the least dense body structures appear *black*, and the more dense structures, which have absorbed the x-rays, appear *white*.

In addition to plain-film radiography, there are many diagnostic x-ray methods. *Fluoroscopy* allows us to study internal body functions, e.g., cardiac motion, peristalsis of bowel. In fluoroscopy, the image is portrayed through an intensifier onto a television monitor. Individual static radiographs can also be taken during this procedure. *Cineradiography* is the recording of successive fluoroscopic images on videotape or motion picture film.

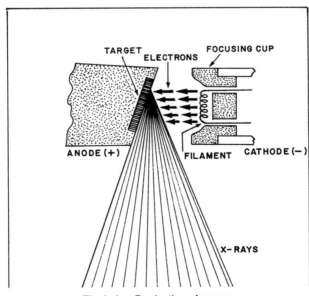

Fig 1–1.—Production of x-rays.

Some x-ray studies involve the use of contrast media, which are substances used to visualize various structures of the body. They can be injected, swallowed, or given as enemas. Examples of contrast media are air, barium sulfate, or organic iodine compounds. The latter two are quite dense and absorb the x-ray beam— hence their usefulness in demonstrating internal structures.

Angiography is the study of blood vessels after contrast has been injected. The contrast medium flowing through the blood vessels of selected organs or masses reveals minute vascular detail.

Radionuclide imaging utilizes a radioisotope-tagged pharmaceutical. When injected, it accumulates in specific tissues and organs, where it emits gamma rays (similar to x-rays) that can be recorded on film or in a computer.

Computed tomography (CT) utilizes an x-ray beam in a rotating carriage to scan a narrow cross-section of the body. Many scans in the same plane are made at different angles. A computer within the CT unit synthesizes the data generated by this process and reconstructs them into images that can be displayed on a television monitor or recorded on disc or tape for later use.

Nuclear magnetic resonance (NMR) is similar to CT in that it uses a computer and scans narrow cross-sections of the body. However, it measures the response of the various chemical components of the body (e.g., hydrogen) to a magnetic field. There is no ionizing radiation.

RADIATION DOSE

The question of the harmful effects of x-rays is frequently raised by concerned parents. Because parents so often express such concern, it is helpful for you to have some basic facts about radiation dosage[2] so that parents can be reassured.

All of us are exposed to approximately 100–150 millirads (mR) per year from the environment (the higher the altitude, the greater the dose). A normal chest examination (two views) exposes the patient to between 10 and 20 mR, while an intravenous urogram imparts approximately 500 mR. Fluoroscopic studies are more radiation-producing than static studies. A barium study of the gastrointestinal tract, for example, exposes the patient to approximately 1,200 mR (1.2 rad). How few millirads cause biologic damage? No one really knows. Therefore, the best policy is to expose a patient to only the amount of radiation that a specific medical problem dictates. However, when a child's medical condition warrants taking a number of radiographs, the benefits of the diagnostic study outweigh any risks. It is extremely important to stress this fact when talking with parents. You can also help to allay anxiety by pointing out the many precautions taken to minimize dangerous ionizing radiation to both patients and staff. X-ray room walls and floors are all shielded, and machines are routinely inspected to assure continued accurate functioning. As pediatric radiologists, we are specially trained to reduce radiation doses for children. We tailor the examination to fit a child's specific problem and use special equipment (105-mm spot films) and procedures (e.g., shielding the reproductive organs).

PROPER UTILIZATION OF RADIOGRAPHS

The major problem of proper utilization is overutilization. Patients are often subjected to excessive radiation per film or an excessive number of films per examination—two factors that can be controlled by the radiologist. With the proper equipment, correct collimation, filtration of the beam, fast screens, cassettes and films, the radiation dose per exposure decreases. One of the most important factors in decreasing excessive radiation per film is a properly trained radiologic technician who will get the correct exposure without having to repeat procedures needlessly.

The number of films per examination must be carefully determined by the radiologist. When a child is having a follow-up examination for urinary abnormalities, for example, a three-film urogram may be appropriate, while another child who is having a first examination may require six films. Similarly, the number of films obtained for a pediatric barium enema differs from that of an adult because of the different nature of the diseases involved.

The most important aspect, however, of proper utilization is appropriate ordering of examinations. The clinician's lack of knowledge of the *capabilities* and *limitations* of a radiographic procedure, overdependence on the radiographic rather than the clinical picture, and the use of radiography as a screening procedure can all lead to many unnecessary films. Moreover, in some areas, especially the emergency room, the patient's demand for a specific procedure—an "x-ray"—adds to further improper utilization.

Finally, our litigious society forces all of us—in our practice of defensive medicine—to order too many radiographs.

- A skull film for insignificant trauma
- Multiple chest films for a child recovering from pneumonia
- A routine preoperative chest film
- Abdominal series and barium studies for nonspecific abdominal pain
- Repeated skeletal studies for children whose bone syndromes have been already diagnosed
- Skeletal surveys for metabolic disease when one film of the extremity will suffice
- Daily films of patients in the intensive care unit whether they need them or not

The best way to decrease such overutilization is to have a pediatric radiologist screen all procedures. In many departments, a radiologist approves all procedures involving contrast media, but it is often impractical—if not impossible—for a radiologist to screen every examination. However, educating pediatricians can markedly improve their ordering of radiographic procedures. When appropriate, the pediatric radiologist can also suggest the newer, noninvasive modalities, such as diagnostic ultrasound, to supplant some radiographic procedures with ionizing radiation.

The radiologist who examines children has a multifaceted role (1) as a *consultant* determining the appropriate examination(s) and the number of films necessary (thereby determining radiation dose), (2) as a member of the *health care team* interpreting films, and (3) as a *teacher* of his clinical colleagues.

SUGGESTED READING

1. Christensen E.E., Curry T.S. III, Dowdey J.E.: *An Introduction to the Physics of Diagnostic Radiology*, ed. 2. Philadelphia, Lea & Febiger, 1978.
2. *Radiation Protection in Pediatric Radiology.* NCRP Report 68. Washington, National Council on Radiation Protection and Measurements, 1981.

CHAPTER **2**

Chest Examinations in Children

THE CHEST FILM is the most frequently ordered pediatric radiographic examination. However, because you look at so many chest radiographs, familiarity may create a false sense of security rather than expertise. A thorough, detailed, systematic approach to the radiographic evaluation is crucial for anyone dealing with children. In this chapter, we discuss the general diagnostic principles and approach; the specifics of chest examinations for neonates and infants are reviewed in Chapter 3. This chapter also stresses those areas where the approach to the pediatric chest radiograph differs from the adult film (e.g., technical problems, unique anatomical and pathological conditions).

TECHNICAL FACTORS

Technical problems in pediatric radiology are largely caused by uncooperative children. The young patients are not feeling well, the environment is strange, and they may, as a result, be quite frightened. Your preliminary evaluation of the chest radiograph should assess these technical factors:
1. The degree of inspiration—lung volume
2. The position of the patient—extent of rotation and posture of the patient
3. How the exposure was made—anterior-posterior or posterior-anterior and appropriate tube-film distance
4. Adequacy of the exposure

LUNG VOLUME

The radiographic examination of the chest begins with frontal and lateral roentgenograms taken after deep inspiration. The degree of inspiration—i.e., the lung volume—will, in general, determine what you see on the film. The answers to the questions in Table 2–1 determine whether or not adequate lung volume was obtained.

If the child has taken a shallow breath, the heart may appear enlarged, the vessels may coalesce to give a false impression of an infiltrate, especially in the region of the bases and hila, and sometimes the radiograph has a hazy quality due to the influx of blood and lack of aerated lung.

Hyperexpansion of the lungs—pathological increase in lung volume or air-trapping—is involuntary, and the changes of hyperexpansion listed in Table 2–1 should be visible on both frontal and lateral films. Figures 2–1 through 2–4 demonstrate the differences between the normal radiograph and the ones where inspiration is either pathologically increased or suboptimal. Can you pick out the optimal radiograph?

4

TABLE 2–1.— Determining Lung Volume

QUESTION	ANSWER
How much of the heart projects below the dome of the diaphragm on the frontal view?	*Greater than* ⅓: expiratory effort; not enough air in the lungs *Less than* ⅓: good inspiratory effort; normal amount of air *None:* may be hyperexpanded; too much air
On the frontal view, are the domes of the diaphragm flat?	*No:* very domed; expiratory effort *Rounded:* good inspiratory effort *Yes:* flat; good or may be possibly too great a lung volume
Are the hemidiaphragms vertically oriented on the lateral?	*No:* horizontally oriented; expiratory effort *Yes:* vertically oriented; good or possibly increased lung volume
Which anterior rib crosses the diaphragm on the frontal film? (Remember that the anterior ribs move more than the posterior ribs on good inspiration.)	*3d or 4th:* expiratory effort *5th or 6th:* inspiratory effort *7th or lower:* good or possibly too great a lung volume
On the lateral view, is there a triangle of air behind the heart?	*No:* expiratory effort (except if large heart) *Yes:* inspiratory effort
Are the lungs black or white on the frontal film?*	*Black:* air filled; inspiratory †*White:* not air filled; expiratory

*Lung density is influenced by exposure. See text, p. 13.
†At times there may be a good lung volume, but the lungs are "white." This white appearance is caused when the child holds its breath while simultaneously pushing against the closed glottis, thus increasing intrathoracic pressure.

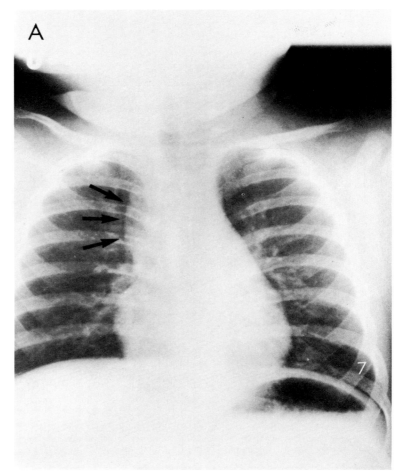

Fig 2–1.—Inspiratory chest. **A,** frontal examination reveals a normal lung volume. The criteria for a normal lung volume are: (1) less than one third of the heart is projected below the hemidiaphragm; (2) the diaphragm is rounded, and the seventh anterior rib intersects the diaphragm; and (3) the lungs are air filled (black). This is a properly positioned, nonrotated film as evidenced by (1) comparative anterior ribs equidistant from the pedicles, (2) medial aspects of the clavicles symmetrically positioned, (3) the carina approximating the right pedicles, and (4) no difference in aeration between the two sides. This film was taken with the patient erect, as shown by the air-fluid level in the stomach. The right lobe of the thymus is prominent *(arrows)* but entirely within normal limits. *(continued.)*

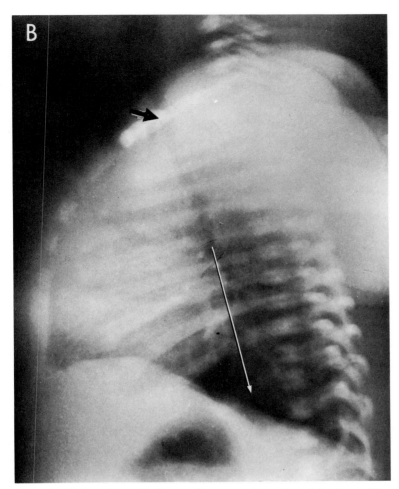

Fig 2–1 (cont.).—B, lateral examination confirms normal aeration of the lungs. The normal triangular air space is seen behind the heart bounded by the heart anteriorly, the diaphragm inferiorly and the vertebrae posteriorly. The patient is not rotated, as the spinous processes of the vertebrae are seen. An air-fluid level in the stomach attests to the erect position of the patient. The airway can be seen from the oropharynx to the carina and is not bowed forward. Note the normal indentation at the thoracic inlet *(black arrow).* The anterior mediastinal space above the heart contains normal thymic tissue. The heart does not project behind an imaginary line extending from the anterior tracheal wall inferiorly.

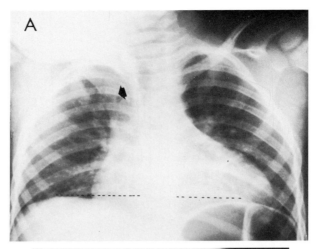

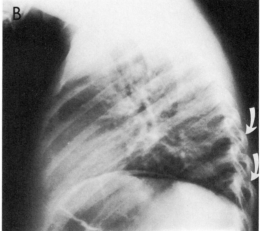

Fig 2–2.—Expiratory chest. **A,** normal frontal film taken during expiration, i.e., (1) more than one third of the heart projects below the diaphragmatic margins; (2) hemidiaphragms are domed, and the fourth anterior rib crosses the diaphragmatic margin; and (3) the lungs are not well aerated (not black). The patient is rotated, as shown by (1) asymmetric comparable ribs in relationship to the pedicles and (2) asymmetric position of the clavicles. The right clavicle is to the right of the sternum *(arrow)*, and (3) the right lung does not appear as well aerated (black) as the left. **B,** expiratory lateral film shows the loss of air space behind the heart. The ribs *(arrows)* are seen but not the spinous processes of the vertebrae, indicating rotation.

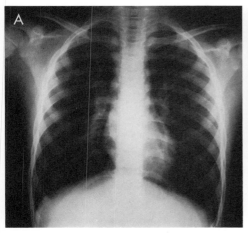 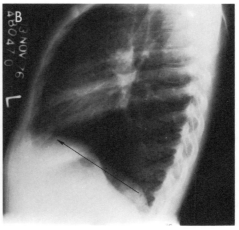

Fig 2–3.—Hyperexpanded frontal and lateral radiographs. **A,** frontal view. The entire heart is projected above the diaphragm, the hemidiaphragms are flattened, and the lungs are quite black— yet the film is not overexposed. **B,** lateral view. The hemidiaphragms are vertically oriented *(arrow),* and there is a very large air space both behind and in front of the heart. Remember, hyperexpansion is involuntary and is caused by air trapping. It must be seen on both frontal and lateral projections.

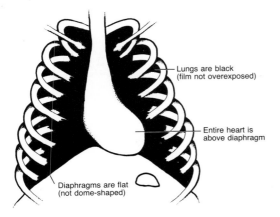

— Lungs are black
(film not overexposed)

— Entire heart is
above diaphragm

Diaphragms are flat
(not dome-shaped)

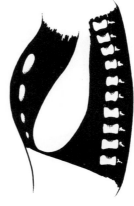

Fig 2–4.—The hyperexpanded chest.

POSITION OF THE PATIENT

The position of the patient is determined by rotation and posture (lying, sitting, or standing).

The child's *posture* is important. When the patient is supine, the vascular supply to the upper and lower lobes is equal since gravity has no effect. When the child is sitting or standing, gravity plays a significant role, and the upper-lobe vessels are less distended than the lower-lobe vessels (one-third to two-thirds size). You can tell an erect film by looking at the air-fluid level in the stomach and at changes in the pulmonary vasculature (see Fig 2–1).

Rotation of a child is determined by the answers to the questions in Table 2–2. Figures 2–5 and 2–6 show the parameters that determine rotation, while Figure 2–7 exemplifies the posture of the patient, showing supine and erect films. Compare these figures with Figure 2–1.

TABLE 2–2.—DETERMINING ROTATION

QUESTION	ANSWER
On the frontal film, are the anterior ribs equidistant from the ipsilateral pedicles?	*No:* rotated patient *Yes:* straight patient
Are the medial aspects of the clavicles symmetrical in relation to the midline on the frontal view?	*No:* rotated patient *Yes:* straight patient
What is the position of the carina in relation to the right pedicles on the frontal film?	*To the left of the right pedicles:* patient is rotated, or another abnormality is present *Approximating the right pedicles:* patient is straight
Is one lung blacker than the other on the frontal view?	*Yes:* patient is rotated, or abnormality is causing localized difference in aeration *No:* straight patient
On the lateral view, are the ribs seen posteriorly?	*Yes:* rotated patient *No:* straight patient

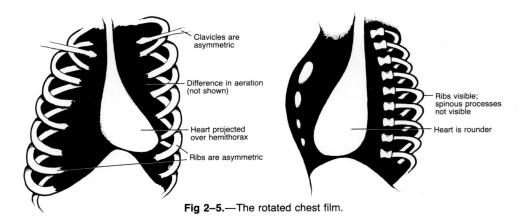

Fig 2–5.—The rotated chest film.

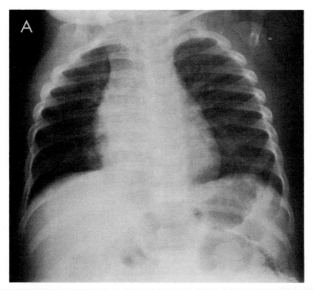

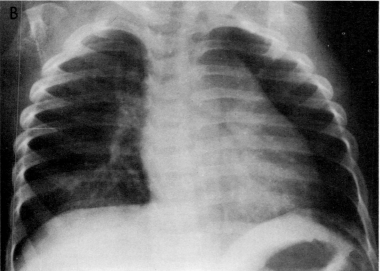

Fig 2–6.—Examples of rotated films. **A** and **B** are films of two different children rotated in opposite directions. In each, can you find the four parameters for estimating rotation? In **A,** to which side is the patient rotated? In **B,** to which side is the patient rotated? (Answers in Appendix 2.)

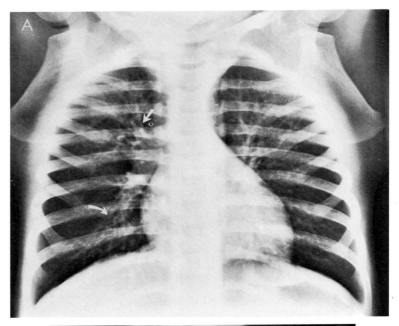

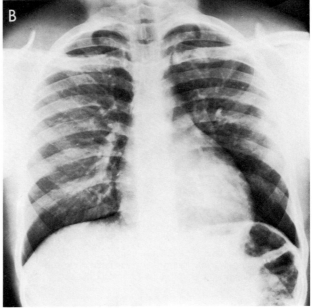

Fig 2–7.—Effect of patient position and tube target distance. **A,** patient in supine position, with approximately 46 inches between the x-ray tube and the film. Upper-lobe vessels *(arrows)* are equal in size to those of the lower lobe *(arrows).* The heart is only minimally magnified. **B,** patient is erect and 6 feet from the x-ray tube. *(continued.)*

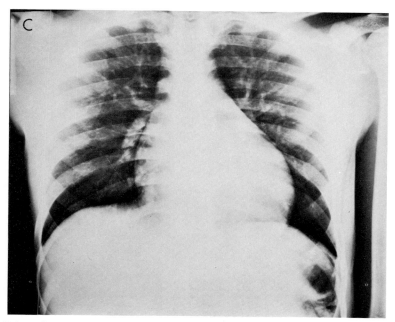

Fig 2–7 (cont.).—C, supine film, tube 40 inches from the film. Note magnification of the heart and mediastinum, and the equally prominent vascularity in both upper and lower lungs.

METHODS OF FILM EXPOSURE

The third major technical factor to keep in mind is how the film was obtained. Greater magnification occurs when structures, e.g., the heart, are farther from the film. When the x-ray beam passes through the patient from back to front (a posterior-anterior [PA] projection), the heart is closer to the film and is less magnified. Conversely, if the x-ray beam enters the patient's chest, passes through the back and onto the film (an anterior-posterior [AP] projection), the magnified heart and great vessels may give the impression of cardiomegaly. This is a common problem with portable chest films, which are taken in the AP direction.

Another important factor in magnification is the distance of the x-ray tube from the film. Routinely, portable films are exposed 40 inches from the tube, adding to the magnification. Figures 2–7 and 2–8 show the principles of magnification and the criteria for recognizing how a film was obtained.

ADEQUACY OF EXPOSURE

Be sure that the film is properly exposed. You can tell this on the frontal film by examining the vertebral column *behind the heart.* If you can see the detailed spine through the heart and can also see the pulmonary vessels behind the heart, the exposure is correct. If you see *only* the spine but not the pulmonary vessels, the film is too dark *(overexposed).*

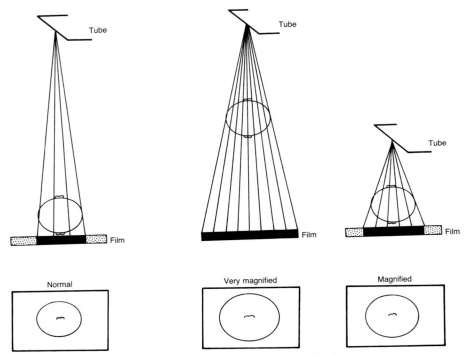

Fig 2–8.—Tube-film distance and magnification.

INTERPRETING THE FILM—THE RADIOLOGIST'S CIRCLE

Anyone can glance at a pediatric chest film, and with very little training identify obvious abnormalities—right? WRONG! It takes most radiologists years to get into the habit of reading a chest radiograph properly. Let's face it; anyone ordering a chest film is going to look at the heart and lungs, but radiologists look first at the nonpulmonary areas: (i.e., the abdomen, bones, soft tissues, and airway) to be sure they don't miss any abnormality. Only then will they go to the cardiopulmonary anatomy.

A good habit to develop is to make an imaginary circle on the film so as to dispense with all the noncardiopulmonary areas. Begin at the corner where the patient information is. Check the name, date, and especially the left or right marker. Nothing is more embarrassing than missing dextrocardia with abdominal situs inversus because you didn't look for the marker and therefore put the film up wrong. An easy way to complete the circle is to go from the name tag to the markers to the ABC's of the film: A = abdomen, B = bones and soft tissues, C = chest (airway, mediastinum, lungs, and diaphragm).

REED'S RULE #1—On every chest film, read the abdominal portion
as you would read an abdominal film.*

---

*Throughout this text, we have included these fundamental concepts, which are used daily in the teaching sessions of Joseph O. Reed, M.D.

ABDOMEN

Evaluate the abdomen (regardless of how little you may be able to see) on every chest film, and note whether the stomach bubble is on the left and the liver on the right. Look specifically for calcifications, such as gallstones or pancreatic stones. Is the bowel distended? Are there air-fluid levels? (Is this an erect film?) Can you see free intraperitoneal air or fluid? Now look at Figure 2–9 with these clues in mind; on every chest film, look at the abdomen as if you were reading an abdominal film.

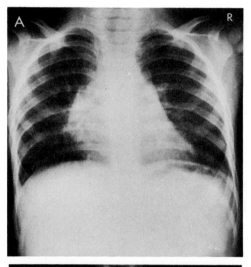

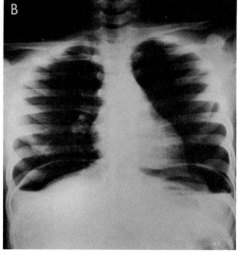

Fig 2–9.—Can you find the abnormality? (Look at the films; then read on.) **A,** film of a 12-month-old-boy. No, the film is not labeled incorrectly. The patient has dextrocardia and abdominal situs inversus. **B,** 9-year-old girl with abdominal pain. Free air is seen beneath the diaphragm. (Note how you see both sides.) The patient has a perforated viscus.

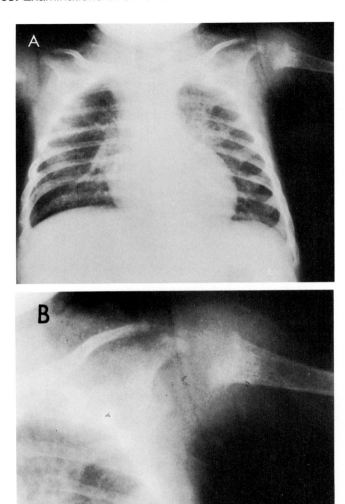

Fig 2–10.—A, look at the *entire* film. This 5-month-old infant had severe renal failure. This frontal view of the chest reveals that, while the heart size is normal, there is a density (in this case, pneumonia) in the left upper lung. However, the bones are indistinct and irregular suggesting severe rachitic changes best seen in the left humerus. The child has renal osteodystrophy. Did you look at the bones? (See Chap. 7.) **B,** cone down view of left shoulder.

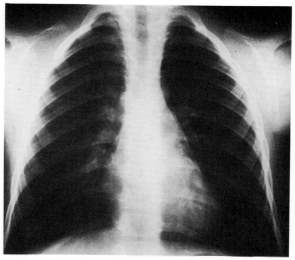

Fig 2–11.—A 9-year-old boy with a cough. (Look at the film; then read on.) Frontal chest film reveals the heart and lungs to be normal, but there is something missing—the clavicles. This patient has cleidocranial dysostosis.

BONES AND SOFT TISSUES

You will often be able to scan portions of the arms, shoulders, ribs, sternum, and mandible, as well as cervical, thoracic, and lumbar vertebrae. Be alert for fractures, congenital abnormalities, bone destruction, or other signs of disease. It is very embarrassing to miss absent clavicles on a chest film because you didn't view the bones systematically. This is also a good time to examine the soft tissues of the neck, thorax, and abdomen to detect any swelling, foreign body, calcifications, etc. The soft tissues may reveal multiple artifacts, such as hair braids, buttons, Band-Aids, or redundant skin folds. Soft tissue swelling or subcutaneous calcifications can be clues to systemic disease. By now, you have returned, via your imaginary circle, to the cervical area, and you are ready to inspect the vertebrae. What abnormalities do you see in Figures 2–10 through 2–14? Look at the films and try to make the diagnosis. Then read the captions.

This brings us to the airway and the beginning of the next category, C, the chest.

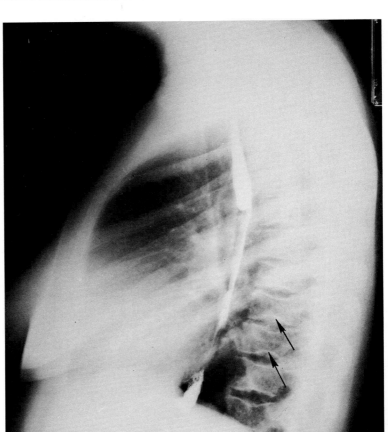

Fig 2–12.—A 17-year-old boy with a cough. On the lateral view, the cortical end plates of most of the thoracic vertebrae are depressed. This patient has sickle cell anemia, and the depressed end plates *(arrows)* are due to infarctions.

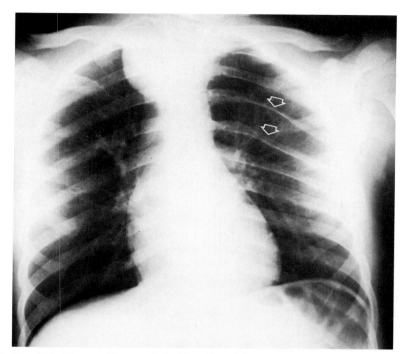

Fig 2–13.—This 12-year-old presented with café au lait spots and scoliosis. Aside from the obvious large mediastinal mass superiorly, there are ribbonlike irregularities of the left fourth through sixth ribs *(arrows)*. The combination of the mediastinal mass, rib changes, and café au lait spots suggests a diagnosis of neurofibromatosis. The chest mass is either an anterior meningocele or a neurofibroma. The ribs are wavy secondary to dystrophic bone and hypertrophied neural tissue in the subcostal groove.

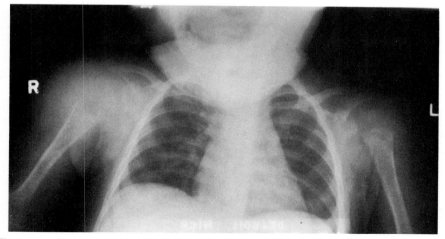

Fig 2–14.—Six-month-old infant with fever of unknown origin. The frontal chest film shows a soft-tissue swelling of the right shoulder and a large lytic lesion of the right humerus. This patient has osteomyelitis.

CHEST (AIRWAY, MEDIASTINUM, LUNGS, DIAPHRAGM)

REED'S RULE #2—Knowledge of anatomy is the key to correct radiographic diagnosis.

AIRWAY

The lateral view of the neck is optimal for evaluating the supraglottic (*supra*, above; *glottis*, vocal cords) airway (Figs 2–15 and 2–16). A proper study is obtained by aligning the top of the film with the top of the patient's ear. The most cephalic portion of the airway is the nasopharynx, which communicates anteriorly with the nares and merges posteriorly into the hypopharynx. For all practical purposes, the borders of the nasopharynx are the soft palate, the uvula, and the adenoid closure. The oropharynx (below the hard and soft palate) leads to the air spaces at the base of the tongue, which are the valleculae. Immediately behind the valleculae is the epiglottis. The oropharynx also merges posteriorly to form the hypopharynx. You can see the palatine tonsils in the lateral walls of the hypopharynx. Inferiorly, the hypopharynx leads to the larynx anteriorly and the esophagus inferiorly and medially. The pyriform sinuses are the most lateral and inferior aspects of the hypopharynx; their inferior margins provide a handy landmark for the level of the vocal cords. It is important, when obtaining a lateral neck examination, to hyperextend the patient's head and neck slightly. This flattens the redundant soft tissues in the retropharyngeal area against the cervical spine.

The frontal radiograph is best for viewing the subglottic airway. The true vocal cords are at the same level as the tip of the pyriform sinuses. Immediately below the glottis is the subglottic region, which is only several millimeters long and merges inferiorly into the proximal trachea (Figs 2–17 and 2–18). Note that the airway is a dynamic system and that an isolated, single film may be quite misleading. Nonetheless, an abnormal configuration of the airway should be pursued in the light of the clinical history. What is the abnormality in Figure 2–19?

REED'S RULE #3—The airway should be visible on all normal chest films.

Figure 2–20 depicts a common pathological state of the airway diagnosed by radiographs of the chest or neck. What is the anatomical abnormality, and what is the disease?

The parameters to evaluate the airway, be it extra- or intrathoracic, are *patency*, *position*, and *size*. You should see the entire airway, from the oral and nasal pharynges to the right and left main-stem bronchi. The walls should be parallel and smooth. However, buckling of the trachea to the right in the lower neck and upper thorax is normal in an infant. The intrathoracic airway is not a midline structure (the carina overlies the right pedicles). What abnormality can you detect in Figure 2–21?

The size of the airway is difficult to ascertain, as it is a dynamic structure that changes in caliber. However, an airway, or a portion thereof, that is consistently narrow demands further investigation.

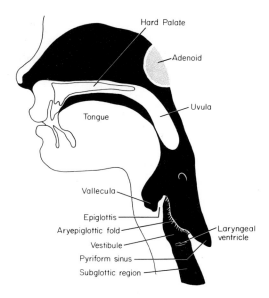

Fig 2–15.—The normal airway, lateral view. (From *Current Problems in Radiology,* vol. 8, Jan.–Feb. 1979. Reprinted with permission of Year Book Medical Publishers.) →

Fig 2–16.—Lateral roentgenogram corresponding to the schematic of Figure 2–15. (From *Current Problems in Radiology,* vol. 8, Jan.–Feb. 1979. Reprinted with permission of Year Book Medical Publishers.) ↓

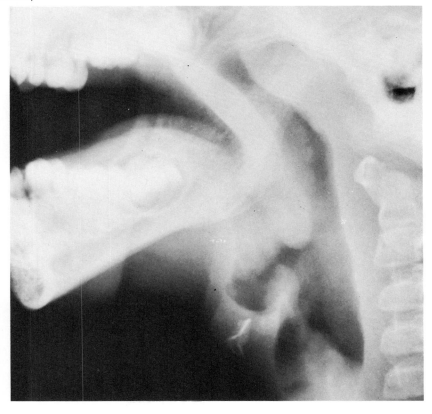

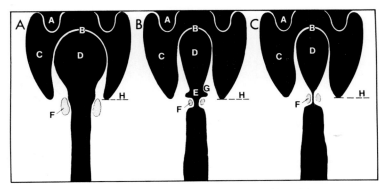

A. Vallecula	E. Larygeal Ventricle
B. Epiglottis	F. True Cords
C. Pyriform Sinuses	G. False Cords
D. Vestibule	H. Tip of Pyriform Sinus – Level of True Cords

Fig 2–17.—Schematic drawings of the frontal airway during various phases of respiration and phonation. (From *Current Problems in Radiology,* vol. 8, Jan.–Feb. 1979. Reprinted with permission of Year Book Medical Publishers.)

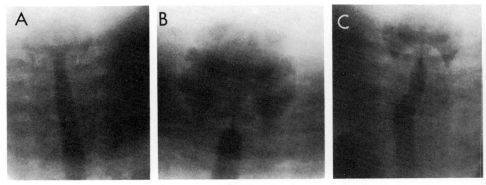

Fig 2–18.—Three frontal radiographs corresponding to the schematics in Figure 2–17.

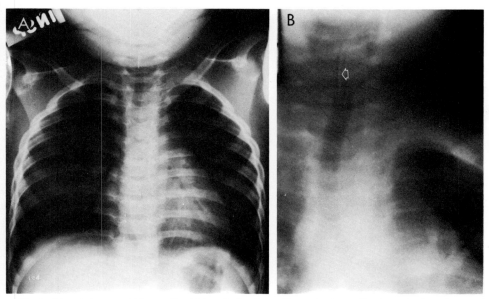

Fig 2–19.—A 1-year-old boy with stridor. **A,** frontal radiograph shows the lungs to be of normal volume and the heart of normal size. The thoracic airway is clearly demonstrated, but there is a density overlying the airway in the cervical region. **B,** magnified high-kilovoltage films show a foreign body in the airway *(arrow).* A piece of eggshell was later removed. (From *Pediatrics* 59:872, 1977. Reprinted with permission.)

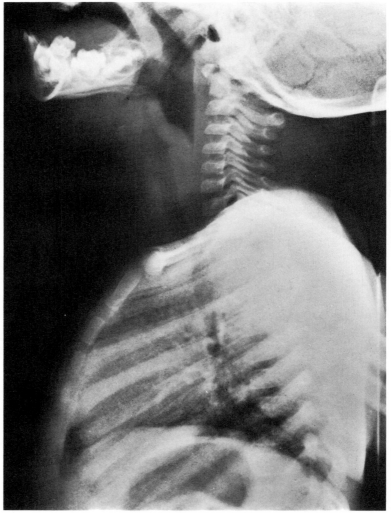

Fig 2–20.—What anatomical abnormality can you see in this examination? (Answer in Appendix 2.)

Fig 2–21.—Six-month-old infant with cough. **A,** frontal radiograph shows the carina pushed to the left. There is a bulge on the right side of the airway. Can you see a normal aortic arch on the left? This is a right aortic arch to the right of the trachea with a right descending aorta *(arrow)* to the right of the spine. **B,** lateral roentgenograph reveals a normal airway. This child had congenital heart disease, tetralogy of Fallot. Many children with this disease have a right aortic arch.　　　　→

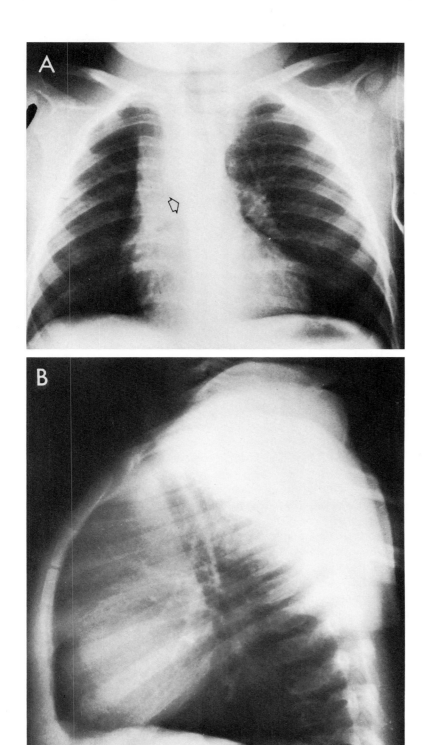

Fig 2–21.

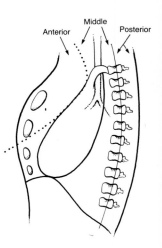

Fig 2–22.—Mediastinum. *Anterior,* the space in front of the heart and great vessels. *Middle,* the space between the anterior and posterior mediastinal components, including heart, airway, esophagus, and lymph nodes. *Posterior,* everything *behind* a line connecting the anterior aspects of the vertebrae, including the vertebrae, neural elements, and paraspinal lymph tissue. (See page 43 for masses typical of these areas.)

MEDIASTINUM

The mediastinum is composed of the thymus, trachea, heart, great vessels, esophagus, lymph nodes, and neural elements. Radiographically, it is separated into the anterior, middle, and posterior compartments (Fig 2–22). In examining the mediastinum, remember

> REED'S RULE #2—*Knowledge of anatomy is the key to correct radiographic diagnosis.*

In the mediastinum, look for *position, size,* and *contour* of the individual components.

THE THYMUS.—One of the major factors that makes pediatric chest x-rays difficult to evaluate is the thymus. It is said that he who masters the thymus has mastered 90% of pediatric chest films because this gland can simulate cardiac enlargement, lobar collapse, pulmonary infiltrates, and mediastinal masses. The thymus is prominent in many children until 4 or 5 years of age. It starts to become a problem when it is still prominent in children over age 5.

The thymus is always anterior in position, which is why the anterior air space on a lateral film appears "full." This is also why it is difficult to diagnose right heart enlargement in a younger child on the basis of fullness of the anterior mediastinum. Since it is such an anterior structure, it is subject to wide variations in position on the frontal chest radiograph. That is, even with the slightest degree of rotation, the thymus may obscure almost the entire right or left lung. To avoid errors in interpretation, check the degree of inspiration and the position of the patient before deciding about unusual densities (Fig 2–23) (see Technical Factors, pp. 4–14).

Thymic size is a major area of concern. The thymus may occupy the entire anterior thorax, entending down to the diaphragm and out to the lateral thoracic wall. It usually shrinks as the child gets older, but thymic remnants can remain even into adulthood. It is a unique organ which also shrinks during periods of stress. It is not unusual to find a small thymus in an obviously sick infant that returns to normal or even "supernormal" size after the infant recovers.

The contour of the thymus is "wavy" because it insinuates itself between the

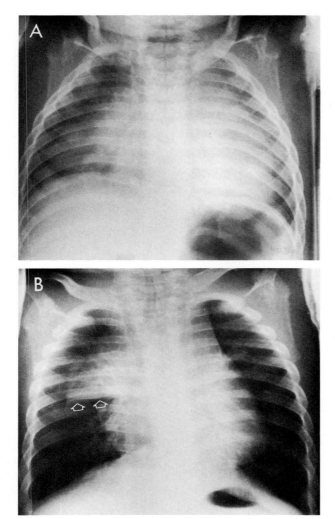

Fig 2–23.—Six-month-old infant with cough. **A,** frontal radiograph shows all the parameters of a film taken during expiration. If you are not acquainted with these criteria, you may interpret this film as showing an infiltrate in both lungs. (See Figure 2–2 for criteria establishing that the film is taken during expiration.) **B,** with a good inspiratory effort, same child shows that the major component of these "infiltrates" was really the thymus which is quite prominent on the right. Notice the thymic sail sign *(arrows).*

anterior ribs. It is a "soft" organ and does not push other mediastinal structures about. Occasionally, fluoroscopy is necessary to decide if the contour of this "mediastinal mass" is indeed wavy and anterior, consistent with a thymus.

THE HEART.—The heart must also be evaluated for *position, size,* and *contour.* Its position is normally in the left hemithorax with a small right thoracic margin.

The appearance of the heart on the frontal film depends greatly on the degree of inspiration and on the size of the thymus. For these reasons, on the lateral roentgenogram, the air space behind the heart and the position of the anterior margin of the trachea play a major diagnostic role. When you draw a line along the anterior

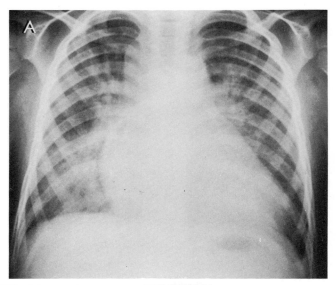

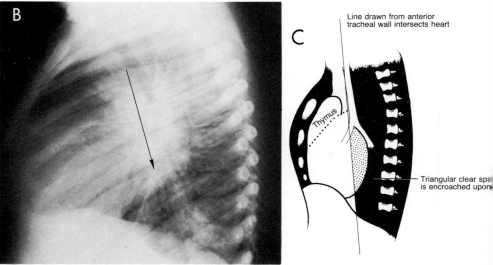

Fig 2–24.—Evaluation of cardiac enlargement on the lateral film. When the heart is behind a line drawn from the anterior tracheal wall to the spine, there is cardiomegaly. In addition, the trachea may be pushed back by a large heart. Frontal **(A)** and lateral **(B)** films of the chest show cardiomegaly with indistinct pulmonary vessels. The vessels in the upper half of the lung are more distinct than those in the lower, due to pulmonary venous congestion causing fluid to leak into the interstitium of the lung, obscuring the pulmonary vessels. A large heart and fuzzy vessels should suggest conges- tive heart failure. **C,** cardiac enlargement, lateral film.

portion of the trachea and project it inferiorly to the diaphragm, it should not in- tersect the heart (Fig 2–24). Additionally, the trachea should not be pushed back against the spine (see Fig 2–1). An enlarged heart will push the trachea back, as will other mediastinal abnormalities. Therefore, if a frontal film shows questionable cardiac enlargement, look at the lateral! If the lateral film is normal, then the heart size is normal as defined by Reed's Rule #4.

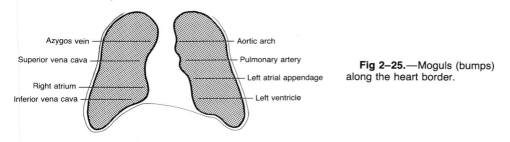

Azygos vein
Superior vena cava
Right atrium
Inferior vena cava
Aortic arch
Pulmonary artery
Left atrial appendage
Left ventricle

Fig 2–25.—Moguls (bumps) along the heart border.

REED'S RULE #4—A mass must be seen in two planes, i.e., if the heart is really large, it must appear large in two planes.

The *contour* of the heart on plain films, in our experience, is not helpful in determining the specific nature of congenital anomalies. Echocardiography and cardiac catheterization are more accurate methods of diagnosing congenital defects. Nonetheless, evaluating the contour of the heart in an older child where the thymus is not a problem can be valuable. In children, the left atrial appendage is not a prominent bulge on the left side because it is usually obscured by even a small thymus. The pulmonary artery, however, may be prominent normally in adolescents (Fig 2–25).

Pulmonary vascular changes, on the other hand, may give a clue to the exact nature of the cardiac disease. Normally one sees pulmonary vessels in the hila and the middle third of the lungs but not in the more peripheral portion. Signs of increased arterial flow include (1) enlarged central vessels, (2) enlarged vessels in the medial third of the lung, and (3) on the erect film, equalization of vessel size between upper and lower lobes. Venous congestion associated with clinical findings of congestive heart failure can be indicated by (1) loss of distinct vessels at the bases (interstitial edema), (2) alveolar filling (pulmonary edema), or (3) right-sided pleural effusion (see Fig 2–24, A).

It is much more difficult to detect *decreased* pulmonary vascularity. Correlating pulmonary vascularity with heart size and the clinical status of the patient (cyanotic vs. acyanotic) is frequently helpful in determining specifics of congenital heart disease.

THE GREAT VESSELS.—The great vessels that are easily identified are the inferior vena cava (on the lateral view) and the aorta (on the frontal film). The position of the trachea is the key to locating the aortic arch (see Fig 2–21). A right aortic arch is often associated with congenital heart disease or vascular ring which presses on both the airway and the esophagus. For this reason, pay special attention to the tracheal air column and the bulges along either side. The right and left pulmonary arteries are easily identified, and the main pulmonary artery is one of the moguls of the left heart border (Fig 2–25). What is the unusual dilatation above the right main-stem bronchus in Figure 2–26?

THE ESOPHAGUS.—This is another structure seen in the mediastinum. It lies in back of the airway and may contain air in younger children. An air-fluid level in the esophagus, however, is always abnormal. Since esophageal problems may man-

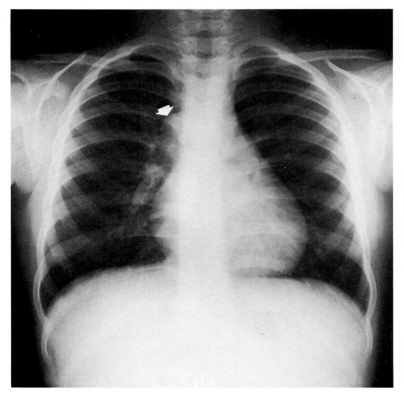

Fig 2–26.—What is the unusual dilatation *(arrow)* above the right main-stem bronchus? In this 4-year-old asymptomatic female (who had the misfortune to have her chest radiographed), a bulge was noted in the junction of the right main-stem bronchus and trachea. It did not pulsate, nor did it affect the esophagus. It was not seen on the lateral film. At ultrasonic examination, the abdominal vena cava was found to be atretic, leaving just a suprahepatic vena cava. The mass is the azygos vein, which returns blood from the abdomen to the heart. This condition is called azygos continuation of the inferior vena cava.

ifest as cardiorespiratory symptoms, a barium swallow is a valuable diagnostic examination in cases of unexplained respiratory disease (Fig 2–27).

> REED'S RULE #5—An esophagram must be done on any child with unexplained respiratory disease.

LYMPH NODES.—Mediastinal lymph nodes are not visible unless they are enlarged.

LUNGS

Let's review the anatomy of the lungs (Fig 2–28). The upper and middle right lobes are separated by the minor fissure frequently seen in a normal chest radiograph. The middle and lower lobes on the right and the upper and lower lobes on the left are separated by the oblique, or major, fissure. These can often be seen on the lateral film. The pulmonary vessels are easily seen branching in the inner two-thirds of the lung. Most of the time, the right hilum is lower than the left; it is never higher. The major bronchi are seen centrally because of the density of the

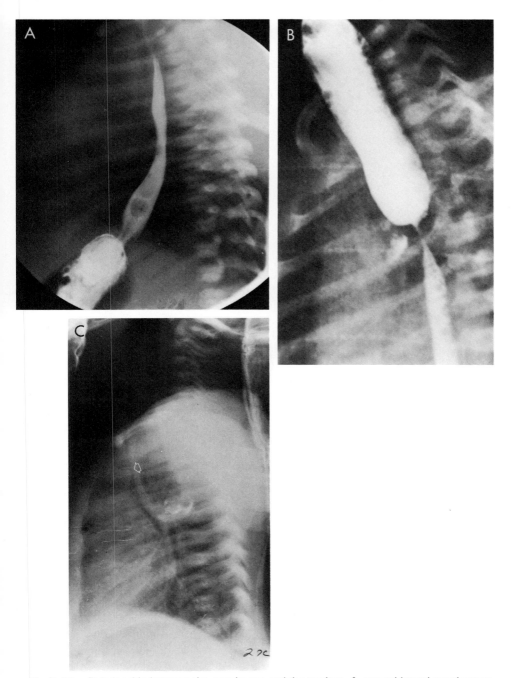

Fig 2–27.—Relationship between the esophagus and the trachea. **A,** normal lateral esophagram. Note the normal trachea and esophagus and their relationship. **B,** lateral view of a child with esophageal stricture. **C,** after the barium has passed through, residual barium remains. Note how the dilated esophagus (now filled with air) compresses the trachea *(arrow).*

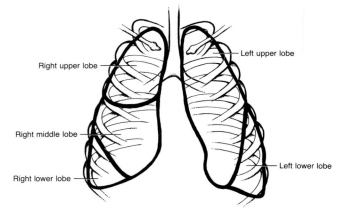

Fig 2–28.—Schematic drawing of lobar anatomy, including fissures.

mediastinum surrounding these air-filled bronchi; they cannot be seen peripherally. There are few lung markings in the peripheral third of the lung. Normally, the pleura is not visible in the lower lobes. The hemidiaphragms change contour with respiration but are nicely dome-shaped on both frontal and lateral films.

Because the lungs are air filled, they offer sharp contrast to the soft-tissue density of the heart and diaphragm, whose margins are quite sharp (see Fig 2–1). If the margins are fuzzy or obliterated, the lung adjacent to these margins is abnormal (the silhouette sign).

COMMON PATHOLOGIC CONDITIONS

HYPEREXPANSION

Hyperexpansion of the lungs results from "air trapping," i.e., the air cannot exit as rapidly as it enters. This may be caused by any functional or organic airway obstruction. Radiologically, hyperexpansion is manifested by flattening or inversion of the diaphragm, widening of the rib interspaces, and larger clear spaces in front and in back of the heart. The heart itself may be compressed and reduced in transverse diameter. The lungs may appear darker than normal, but check that the film was not overexposed (see Fig 2–3). In general, it looks as if the child took a very deep breath when you know he is too young to have followed the technician's instructions. You must see air-trapping on both frontal and lateral views.

When hyperexpansion occurs chronically, cor pulmonale may result. Hyperexpansion may be unilateral or bilateral. Some common causes of *bilateral* hyperexpansion are (1) asthma, (2) bronchiolitis, and (3) cystic fibrosis. Isolated hyperexpansion of one or two lobes *unilaterally* is commonly found in children who have a foreign body or hilar nodes compressing the bronchus. Because of unilateral hyperexpansion, the mediastinum may be shifted. In addition, unilateral hyperexpansion may result from atelectasis or collapse of the contralateral segment of lung (Fig 2–29). Recognizing unilateral hyperexpansion of lung is extremely important in pediatrics because children frequently aspirate foreign material (see Fig 2–29).

> *REED'S RULE #6—In unilateral hyperexpansion of the lungs, you must see how the air moves. Mediastinal position is critical to this determination.*

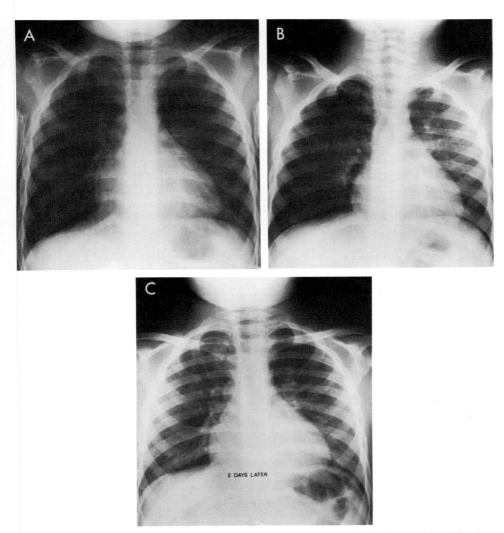

Fig 2–29.—A 3-year-old who started choking after eating peanuts. **A,** inspiratory frontal film has subtle changes: the right lung is hyperexpanded and blacker than the left, although there is no mediastinal shift. **B,** expiratory film reveals that air did not leave the right lung; it remains trapped during the expiratory phase of respiration. The mediastinum is shifted to the left (the left lung has gone through expiration properly). **C,** 2 days after a peanut was removed from the right main-stem bronchus, the expiratory film shows no difference in aeration.

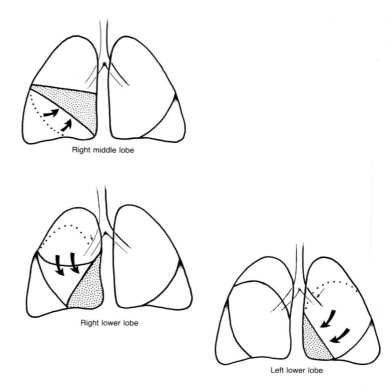

Right middle lobe

Right lower lobe

Left lower lobe

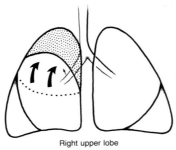

Right upper lobe

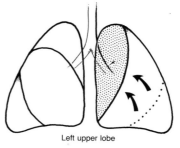

Left upper lobe

Fig 2–30.—Lobar collapse. Note trachea *(small arrow)* and fissure *(large arrow)* shift.

The movement of air within a lung can be visualized by various procedures such as (1) inspiratory and expiratory radiographs (mediastinal position), (2) fluoroscopy of the chest (mediastinal position and diaphragmatic motion), (3) decubitus films (the down side is the "expiratory" side of the radiograph). With these maneuvers, you should be able to see when air in the abnormal side does not move properly (see Fig 2–29).

If there is too much air in one hemithorax, be sure there are lung markings within the area; you might be missing a pneumothorax. It is mandatory to identify the visceral-pleural margin.

LOBAR COLLAPSE

It is often helpful to think of the lobes of the lungs as being attached at the hila as if they were a fan. When these lobes collapse, they still retain their hilar attachment, and the other lobes often expand to compensate. The patterns of lobar collapse are identified in two ways—by seeing the collapsed lobe in a recognizable pattern and by noticing subtle shifts of intrathoracic structures and loss of normal roentgenologic borders (silhouette sign) (Figs 2–30 and 2–31). Five questions should be asked when you see a density that appears to be a lobar collapse:
1. To which side is the mediastinum shifted?
2. In what directions are the major and minor fissures deviated?
3. What normal structures are silhouetted?
4. Is the hilum shifted up or down?
5. Is the diaphragm elevated? (see Figs 2–30 and 2–31.)

A common cause of lobar collapse in children is mucus plugging in postoperative and asthmatic patients. Foreign bodies must also always be looked for by carefully examining the right and left main-stem bronchi. Masses such as lymph nodes (tuberculosis, other infections, or lymphoma) or extrinsic masses, such as bronchogenic cysts, can also cause lobar collapse.

PULMONARY DENSITIES

A pulmonary density may be caused by (1) pneumonic consolidation, (2) atelectasis, (3) neoplasm, or (4) a localized collection of fluid. Sometimes, densities are indistinguishable. In fact, two processes often are co-existent. When discussing this problem with colleagues, beware of the word "infiltrate." It has come to mean a pneumonic process, but some radiologists use it with atelectasis or edema in mind.

Densities within the alveolar space frequently show air bronchograms, which occur when air within the bronchi is seen against a background of airless lung or fluid-filled alveoli. Most alveolar densities are confluent and larger than individual vessels. Any material, such as pneumonic consolidation or fluid from congestive heart failure, may be manifest by alveolar air space density. In diseases such as viral pneumonia and tuberculosis, edema or pus in the interstitium of the lung creates discrete linear streaks. These "increased interstitial markings" represent peribronchial thickening, atelectasis, fibrosis, and what is commonly termed "the radiologic dirty lung," a common finding in patients with chronic asthma. Remember, "increased interstitial markings" are *signs*, not a specific active disease!

Lobar pneumonia can silhouette the mediastinum, mimicking lobar collapse (Fig 2–32). You will not, however, see mediastinal shift of the same magnitude, nor will there be loss of volume with changes of position of the fissures.

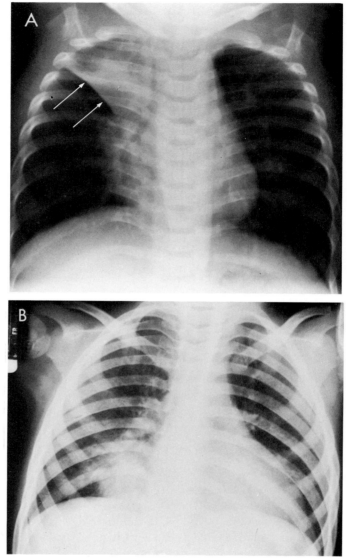

Fig 2–31.—Examples of lobar collapse. **A** and **B,** right upper-lobe collapse with elevation of the minor fissure *(arrows). (Continued.)*

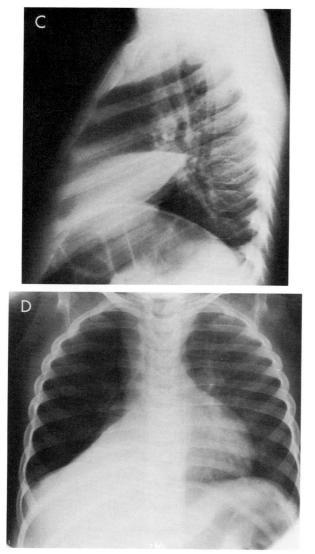

Fig 2–31 (cont.).—C, right middle-lobe collapse with loss of the right heart border (the silhouette sign) and density over the heart on lateral projections. **D,** right lower-lobe collapse. The heart margin is preserved as the right lower lobe collapses toward the midline. *(Continued.)*

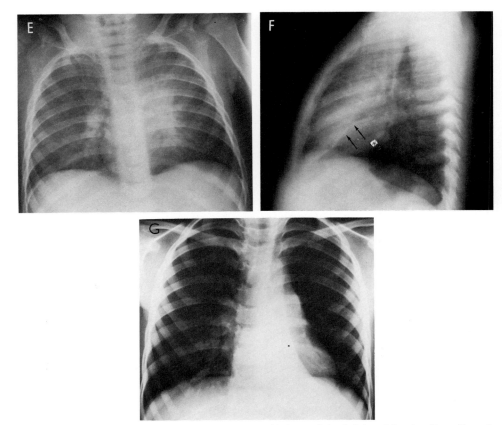

Fig 2–31 (cont.).—E, left upper-lobe collapse with loss of the left heart border (the silhouette sign) and a hazy density over the left upper lung. **F,** lateral film of left upper-lobe collapse. Major fissure *(arrow)* is far anterior to its normal position *(star)*. **G,** left lower-lobe collapse with density behind the heart. The left heart border is not obscured.

The most *overdiagnosed* (nonexistent) pneumonias are: (1) "right lower lobe pneumonia" at the medial lung base, often caused by pulmonary arterial branches seen on a film taken with a poor inspiratory effort and (2) perihilar pneumonia, also caused by slight rotation of the chest and poor inspiration, making the hilar vessels stand out. Be leery of densities in the perihilar regions and the right lower lobe. The most *overlooked* pneumonia is that found in the left lower lobe (see Fig 2–32). This is easily recognized when you remember that the heart should have the same radiodensity throughout. Loss of pulmonary artery visibility or a sudden change from gray to white in any portion of the heart should make you suspicious of retro-cardiac pneumonia. When reading a chest film, train yourself to *look through things.* Also, keep your eye on the left hemidiaphragm; it should be seen as clearly as the right. Any disruption may mean adjacent pneumonia or atelectasis (silhouette sign).

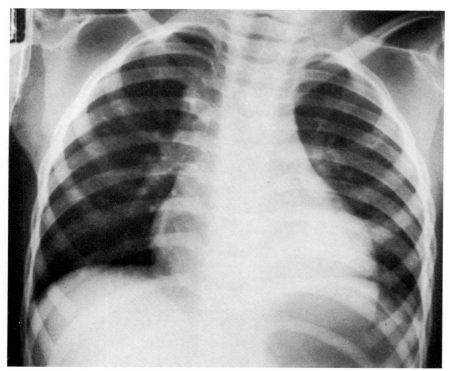

Fig 2–32.—Left lower infiltrate. This 3-year-old has fever and a cough. There is a great deal of density behind the left side of the heart. You can look through the right side of the heart and see the lung and its vascularity. This is not the case on the left—a finding consistent with left lower-lobe pneumonia.

MASSES AND PSEUDOMASSES

A common mass in the lungs of children is really a pseudomass caused by the "round" pneumonia (Fig 2–33). This type of density is sometimes so perfectly round that it simulates a neoplasm. Appropriate treatment is given, and follow-up films are obtained within 10 days to document whether or not the mass disappears. Another pseudomass is caused by loculated fluid in the fissure. Often, this fluid is teardrop-shaped and conforms to the anatomy of the fissure; the density is often sharply demarcated for one-half to three-quarters of its borders (see Fig 2–33).

The common juxta-diaphragmatic pseudomass is due to partial eventration— thinning of the muscles—of the diaphragm; it is most often seen on the right as a "bump" on the diaphragmatic surface. Such a phenomenon is *usually asymptomatic and does not require therapy*, but a large eventration can act as a diaphragmatic hernia, causing mediastinal shifts (Fig 2–34).

True primary neoplasms are uncommon in children. The most common ones are extensions of mediastinal structures or are caused by defects of the diaphragm and are, in fact, extrapulmonary (Fig 2–35). It is appropriate, then, to discuss mediastinal masses in this category. These masses may arise in any of the three components of the mediastinum. The most common posterior mediastinal mass is a neu-

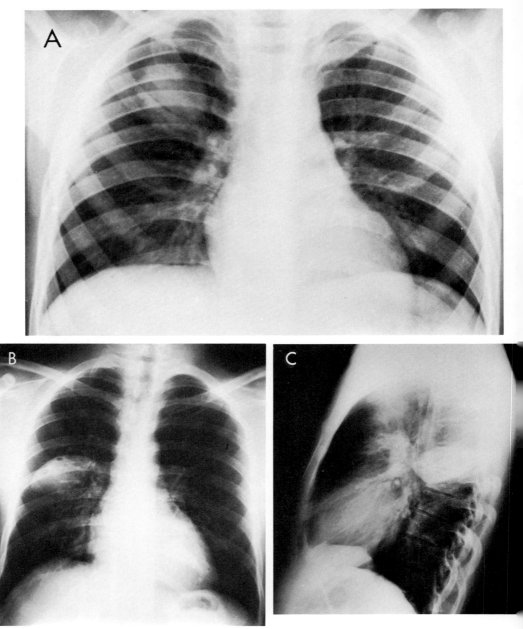

Fig 2–33.—Unusual pulmonary densities. **A,** round pneumonia. Frontal chest film shows a rounded density that might, at first glance, be mistaken for a tumor or metastasis. Antibiotic therapy resulted in a normal chest on subsequent films. **B,** loculated pleural fluid. This child had unexplained fever and cough for 2 weeks after antibiotic therapy for pneumonia. Chest films show an elliptical density on the right. Note how it conforms to the position of the minor fissure. This is characteristic of a loculated effusion (in this case, infected fluid) in the fissure. **C,** lateral film of another child with loculated pleural fluid in the posterior portion of the major fissure.

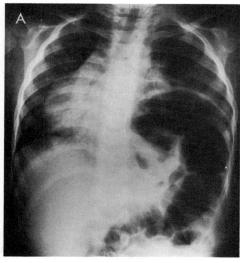
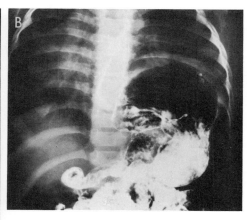

Fig 2–34.—16-month-old with cough. **A,** frontal chest radiograph shows the mediastinum shifted to the right and bowel loops compressing the left lower lung. **B,** barium was given, confirming the intrathoracic location of the stomach and small bowel. At surgery, there was an intact diaphragm, but it was very thin, consistent with a large eventration. When the eventration is this large, it acts as a mass causing the same symptoms as a diaphragmatic hernia.

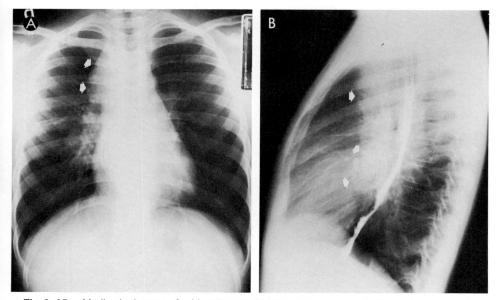

Fig 2–35.—Mediastinal mass. **A,** this 10-year-old has a widened mediastinum. He is too old to have a large thymus and, in fact, has an enlarged right hilum with adenopathy *(arrows)*. **B,** lateral roentgenograph shows the density in the middle mediastinum—a common presentation for a lymphoma *(arrows)*.

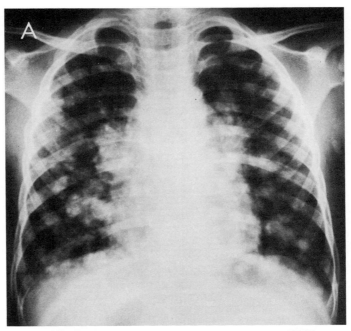

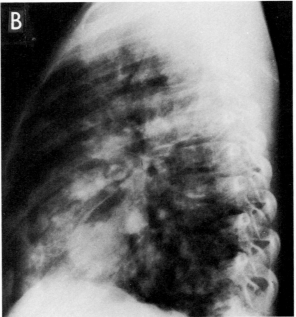

Fig 2–36.—Metastatic lung disease. **A,** this 3-year-old had had a Wilms' tumor removed 7 months previously. There are multiple rounded densities in the chest, and bilateral hilar adenopathy. **B,** lateral film also shows the metastatic tumor nodules as well as some fluid in the major fissure.

rogenic tumor such as a neuroblastoma—ganglioneuroma—or neurofibroma. The hemidiaphragm insets posteriorly at the L1–2 level; therefore, a posterior basilar intrathoracic mediastinal mass may masquerade as an abdominal mass. Remember the normal posterior extent of the chest! Middle mediastinal masses are most commonly of lymphoid origin (e.g., lymphoma), but lesions of any of the other structures of the middle mediastinum—such as esophageal duplication—may occur. The most common anterior mediastinal masses are teratomas, thymomas (in children over 10) and cystic hygromas (with extension down from the neck). True parenchymal masses are frequently due to metastasis such as that from Wilms' tumor (Fig 2–36). Congenital primary masses are discussed in the next chapter.

The outline below is a useful summary of the etiology of mediastinal masses.
  I. Anterior mediastinum
     A. Teratoma
     B. Thymoma
     C. Thyroid
     D. Lymph node enlargement by either infection or malignancy
     E. Cystic hygroma
 II. Middle mediastinum
     A. Esophagus—duplication cysts
     B. Great vessels—aneurysmal dilatation
     C. Hila—enlarged lymph nodes, leukemia, lymphoma, tuberculosis, etc.
     D. Trachea—bronchogenic cysts
III. Posterior mediastinum
     A. Neural tumor—neurofibroma, neuroblastoma, ganglioneuroma
     B. Spinal infectious lesions—tuberculosis (Pott's disease)
 IV. *Tips when viewing mediastinal masses*
     A. Middle mediastinal masses silhouette the heart border and aorta.
     B. Posterior mediastinal masses may spread ribs.

THE PLEURA

Pleural reaction (effusion or thickening) is best indicated by a density between the aerated lung and rib border (Fig 2–37). Thickened pleura, loculated pleural fluid, or empyema appear similar radiographically and cannot always be differentiated by normal radiographic techniques. Decubitus films will demonstrate free-flowing fluid but may not show loculated pleural fluid, viscous empyema, or thickened pleura. An excellent way to detect small amounts of fluid or limited pleural thickening not visible on the frontal film is to look carefully at the posterior lung sulci on the lateral film. Then check the thickness of the pleural line in relationship to each rib; it should be snug against the rib. Fluid can also accumulate beneath the cupola of the lung and can simulate an elevated hemidiaphragm. Such collections are called subpulmonic effusions and are recognized by the laterally shifted "diaphragmatic dome" (see Fig 2–37).

The most common cause of pleural effusion in children is infection, and almost any infection can cause a small pleural effusion. Pleural effusions are also frequently seen in patients with congestive heart failure and chronic renal disease.

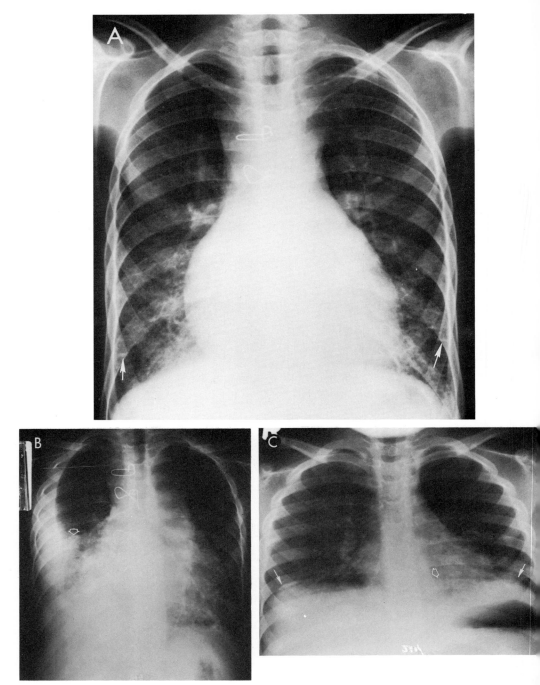

Fig 2–37.—Pleural effusions. **A,** film taken after open-heart surgery. Note the slightly enlarged heart and multiple interstitial lines in both lower lungs. The lines, which are horizontal and extend to the pleura *(arrow),* are called Kerley's B lines. **B,** postpericardiotomy syndrome. A few days after the first film, this child developed an extensive right-sided pleural effusion. The fluid dissected into the region of the minor fissure *(arrow).* **C,** subpulmonic effusion. Careful attention to the apex of the "dome of the diaphragm" shows that it is somewhat laterally situated on both sides of the chest *(arrows).* Note also that the stomach bubble is separated from the "dome of the diaphragm" by a space. There is also a paramediastinal density *(open arrows).* This child had nephritis resulting in a pleural effusion that filled the space below the lung (cupola of lung) and above the diaphragm. This fluid simulates a diaphragmatic border, but, in fact, the diaphragm is not visible.

SUMMARY

A thorough radiographic workup should include the following:
1. Good erect, inspiratory frontal and lateral chest films.
2. Inspiratory and expiratory films (if persistent hyperexpansion or atelectasis is the problem) and/or fluoroscopy of the chest to observe mediastinal shift and diaphragmatic excursion. (Decubitus films may help.)
3. Specialized study of the airway, if the air passage itself needs evaluation (see Chap. 9).
4. An esophagram in any unsuspected airway disease or if a mass is seen on the plain films.

Remember, the chest radiograph can be a very tricky thing. It is easy to get "seduced" by obvious pathology such as a mass density, a large heart, or a large pleural effusion. You must resist the temptation to describe the obvious abnormality and force yourself to do a routine, orderly scan of the chest and "succumb" to the obvious lesion last. This method will help train you to spot more subtle findings, such as a rib fracture. A convenient way to read systematically is to evaluate the technical factors of lung volume, patient position, and the way the film was exposed. Use the radiologist's circle and the ABCs: A = abdomen, B = bones and soft tissues, C = chest (airway, mediastinum, lungs, and diaphragm). Now evaluate Figures 2–38 through 2–42. Approach each one systematically and describe the abnormalities you see. The answers are in the appendix.

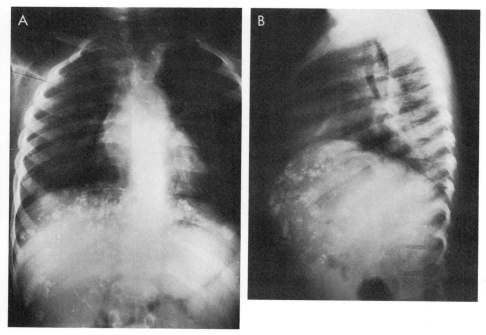

Figure 2–38.—Unusual densities. (See Appendix 2.)

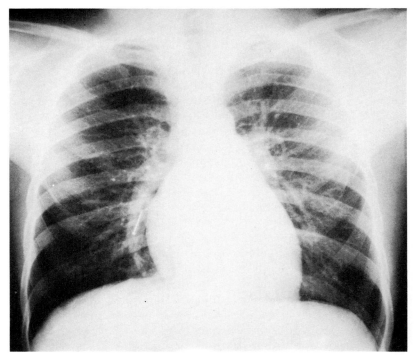

Fig 2–39.—A child with acute onset of respiratory distress. (See Appendix 2.)

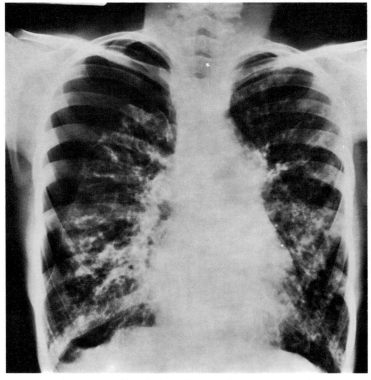

Fig 2–40.—Chronic lung disease. (See Appendix 2.)

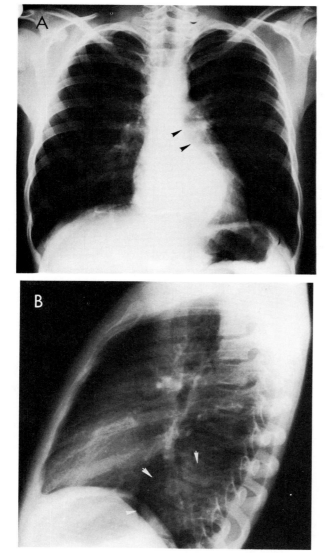

Fig 2–41.—A child with a cough. (See Appendix 2.)

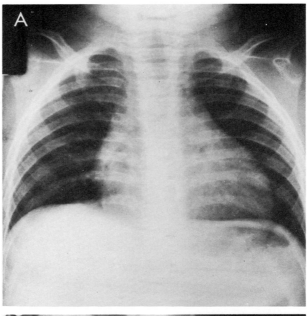

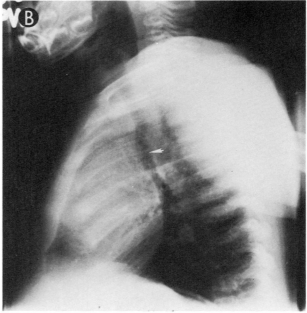

Fig 2–42.—A child with wheezing. *(Continued.)*

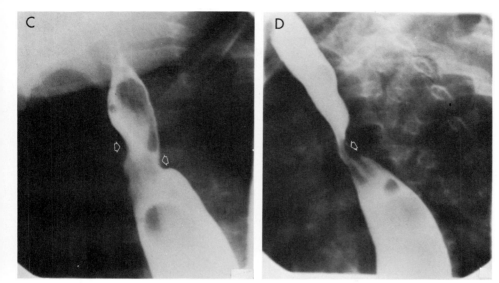

Fig 2–42 (cont.).

SUGGESTED READING

1. Riggs W. Jr.: *Pediatric Chest Roentgenology: Recognizing the Abnormal.* St. Louis, Warren H. Green, Inc., 1979.
2. Felson B., Weinstein A.S., Spita, H.B.: *Principles of Chest Roentgenology—A Program Text.* Philadelphia, W.B. Saunders Co., 1965.
3. Squire L.F.: *Fundamentals of Radiology.* Cambridge, Mass., Harvard University Press, 1964.

CHAPTER **3**

The Chest in the Neonate and Young Infant

RAPID PHYSIOLOGIC CHANGES occur in the first minutes and hours of a newborn's life. The fluid-filled lungs empty of surfactant-rich fluid and fill with air. The circulatory system is dramatically changed when the ductus arteriosus closes. The lungs now receive a major influx of blood, and gaseous exchange occurs. During subsequent weeks, the pulmonary artery pressures fall from near systemic values. This drop in pulmonary vascular resistance permits clinical recognition of left-to-right shunts, such as ventricular septal defects (VSD) and atrial septal defects (ASD).

The newborn infant breathes and cries. Both of these processes fill the lungs and the gastrointestinal tract with air. The lungs fill with air during the first breath. The gastrointestinal tract fills more slowly, and it may take up to 24 hours for gas to reach the rectum (although it occurs by 12 hours in most healthy infants).

The sequence and timing of these expected physiologic and anatomical changes allow the radiologist to detect the infant making an abnormal transition to extrauterine life.

TECHNICAL FACTORS

The method for taking chest films in a neonate differs from that in older children (Chap. 2). The baby remains supine, the film (which is under the baby) is exposed with the x-ray tube above for the anterior-posterior projection. The tube-film distance is 36–40 inches because the equipment must be fixed within the restraints of the isolette and life-support systems (Fig 3–1). A lateral film may be taken by turning the baby onto its side. It may also be taken as a "cross-table lateral," i.e., with the baby supine and the beam directed through the baby's side. The cross-table lateral technique is particularly important when there is a possibility of free air (pneumothorax or pneumomediastinum). Since the child is supine and air rises, air can be seen under the sternum.

On all portable films, there is inherent magnification of mediastinal structures and absence of the effect of gravity on both the pulmonary vascularity and on fluid within the bowel. Why is this important? (Answers in Appendix 2.)

Newborns are unique in other ways: (1) a normal neonate breathes at a rate of 30–50 times per minute and it is therefore more difficult to get a "good inspiratory

Fig 3–1.—Normal chest. **A,** on this frontal supine film the mediastinum is wide, and the lateral margins of the heart are obscured by the thymus. The thymic border is rather indistinct, blending into the lung on the left. **B,** on the lateral view, however, the thymus clearly occupies the anterior mediastinum. There is a triangular air space behind the heart. The heart is entirely anterior to a line drawn from the anterior tracheal wall and is therefore not enlarged. →

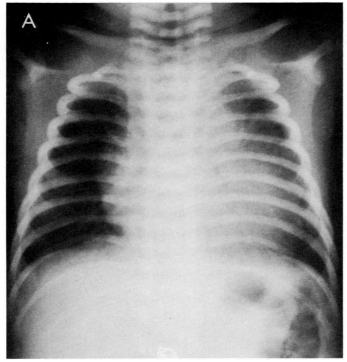

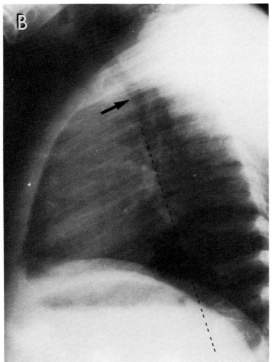

Fig 3–1.

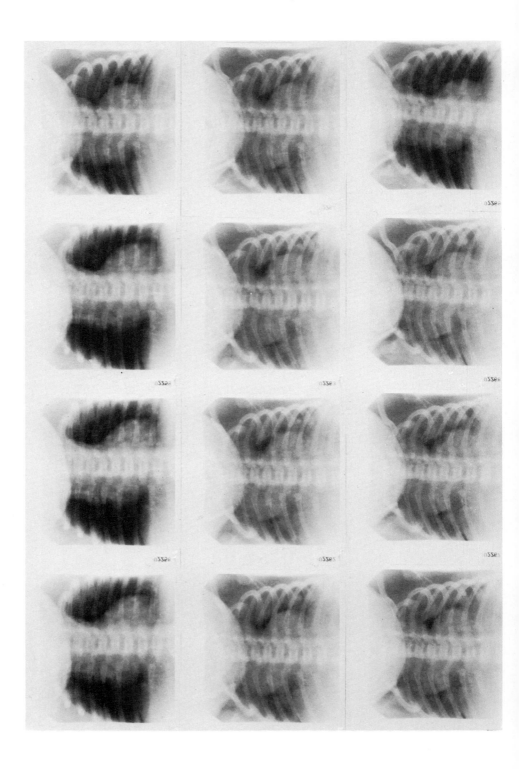

Fig 3–2.—Expiratory-inspiratory sequence. Multiple films obtained during a 12-second interval while this infant with a pneumomediastinum was crying. *Top row*, the heart size is normal, and the lungs are well aerated. *Middle row*, during expiration, the lungs are becoming opaque and filling with blood. The hemidiaphragms are elevated, and a pneumomediastinum outlines the heart. *Bottom row*, by the last film, the patient is again in the inspiratory phase of respiration clearing the lungs. (Courtesy of Walter E. Berdon, M.D., and David H. Baker, M.D., Babies and Children's Hospital, New York.)

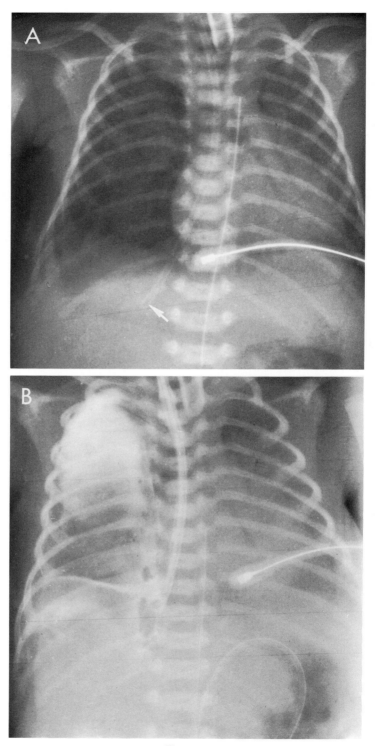

Fig 3–3.

film"; (2) the trachea in the neonate and young infant is "too long" for the contracted chest in expiration, so it buckles; and (3) normal neonates have a large anterior mediastinal mass—the thymus, which is accentuated by the anterior-posterior projection (Fig 3–2).

How, then, does one determine the normal film? What criteria should be used? The approach is the same as that outlined in Chapter 2; lung volume and patient position, i.e., rotation, must be evaluated first (review "Technical Factors" in Chap. 2). The radiologist's circle must be followed; and, since there are multiple films on the sick neonate, strict attention must be paid to the name, date, and time of examination. The ABC approach is important in evaluating the neonatal chest as well.

REED'S RULE #1—On every chest film, read the abdominal portion as you would read an abdominal film.

ABDOMEN

The neonate frequently has an orogastric or nasogastric tube for decompression of a distended stomach and for feeding. Its position must be noted, as it may be in the esophagus (a good situation for aspiration), deep within the small bowel or, worse, extraluminal (Fig 3–3). Venous catheters may be either in an umbilical vein, within the portal venous system, in the inferior vena cava, or in the heart. These venous catheters are seen anteriorly in the umbilical vein and in the liver, while the umbilical artery catheters are posteriorly placed (Fig 3–4). The arterial catheter enters through the umbilical artery, proceeds caudad in the iliac vessels, and then ascends through the abdominal aorta. The catheter course is to the left of the midline.

BONES AND SOFT TISSUES

As one continues in the imaginary circle around the periphery of the film, the bones and soft tissues should be considered as important clues to the well-being of a child. There is little subcutaneous fat in neonates. Usually the soft tissues are quite inconspicuous. However, if there is clinical evidence of hydrops fetalis or hypoproteinemia, the soft tissues exhibit swelling secondary to the edematous state. A rather common soft tissue density is an umbilical clamp and the residual umbilical cord. It may project as a mass in the midabdomen.

Because the neonatal radiograph is the first opportunity you have to detect congenital abnormalities, be sure to check the bones for such abnormalities as hemivertebrae, absence of the clavicles, and fractures secondary to trauma of the birth process. The bones also provide a clue to a possible congenital infection (TORCH infections—*to*xoplasmosis, *r*ubella, *c*ytomegalic inclusion disease, and *h*erpes; some people also include syphilis in this listing).

← **Fig 3–3.**—Perforation by nasogastric tube. **A,** frontal film shows a pneumothorax extending from the mediastinum around the right lung. The tip of the nasogastric tube is in the right side of the chest *(arrow).* **B,** contrast injected into the nasogastric tube spills into the pleural space.

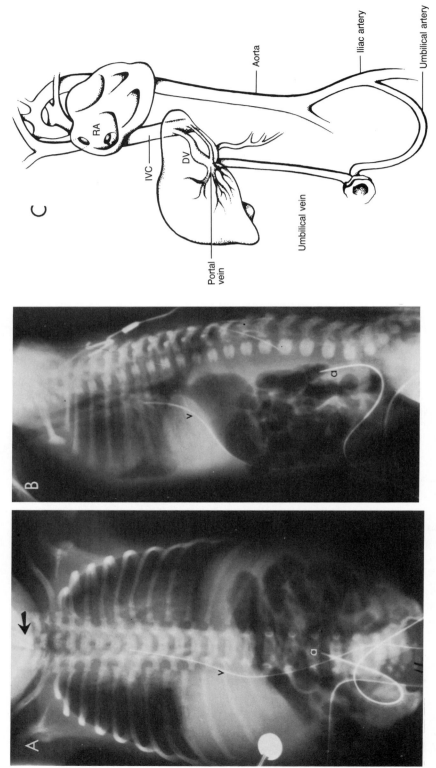

Fig 3–4.—Catheters and tubes. **A,** frontal radiographs of the chest and abdomen reveal the endotracheal tube in the cervical airway (arrow). Two other tubes can be seen: one whose tip ends in a vessel within the abdomen, and one in a vessel within the chest. **B,** the lateral film confirms which tube is arterial (A) and which is venous (V). The anterior catheter starts in the umbilical venosus, into the right atrium. The arterial line dips inferiorly in the iliac artery and then rises posteriorly in the abdominal aorta. **C,** this drawing depicts the anatomy of the umbilical vessels. A catheter in the umbilical vein will cross the portal vein and enter the ductus venosus on its way to the right atrium. The umbilical artery dips down to join the internal iliac artery then the main aorta.

56

CHEST

THE AIRWAY

Again, the parameters used to evaluate the extrathoracic and intrathoracic airway are *patency, position* and *size* (Fig 3–5).

> REED'S RULE #3—*The airway should be visible on all chest films. To examine the airway in detail, it is frequently useful to use your finger as a pointer so that each structure receives your undivided attention.*

Patency.—You should see the airway from the oropharynx and the nasopharynges to the right and left main-stem bronchi. The baby with an obstructed nasopharynx will present with severe respiratory distress because he breathes primarily through the nose.

Position.—Remember that the trachea is *not* a midline structure (the carina projects adjacent to the right pedicles). Buckling of the trachea is normal (see Fig 3–5).

Size.—Airway size is difficult to ascertain, as it is a dynamic structure that changes in caliber. However, if, on all views of the airway, it is persistently small, further investigation is necessary. It is *normal* for neonates and young infants to occasionally have some air in the esophagus (not so in older children).

Sick neonates often require an endotracheal tube. It is crucial to tell the clinician about the relationship of the tube to the carina because these tubes can move. If they slip into the main-stem bronchus on either side (more frequently the right, as it is a straighter drop), obstructive emphysema on one side with atelectasis on the other may occur (Fig 3–6). The ideal position of the endotracheal tube is at the level of the inferior margins of the clavicles.

THE MEDIASTINUM

The heart and mediastinal structures demand attention as to *position, size,* and *contour.*

The *position* is easily determined on a nonrotated film. The aortic arch frequently cannot be seen in a neonate, and its position must be inferred by the position of the carina. On a normal study, the carina overlies the right pedicles, and the aortic arch is therefore positioned on the left. Similarly, a right-sided aortic arch may be inferred if the position of the carina is midline or to the left. A right aortic arch should alert the physician to the possibility of congenital heart disease and/or a vascular ring.

The thymus constitutes the major portion of the mediastinal silhouette in a normal newborn (see Fig 3–1). It may extend from the lung apex to the diaphragmatic surfaces, be insinuated into the minor fissure on the right (giving a "sail sign" or "spinnaker sign"), be bilaterally symmetrical or predominantly one-sided. The normal thymus is situated in the anterior mediastinum and never "pushes" on the airway or any other intrathoracic structures. Because the thymus is so ubiquitous and large, evaluating cardiac size becomes more difficult in the neonate and young infant (the thymus may be seen in some children up to the age of 4 to 5 years).

Size is the second parameter used in evaluating the mediastinal silhouette.

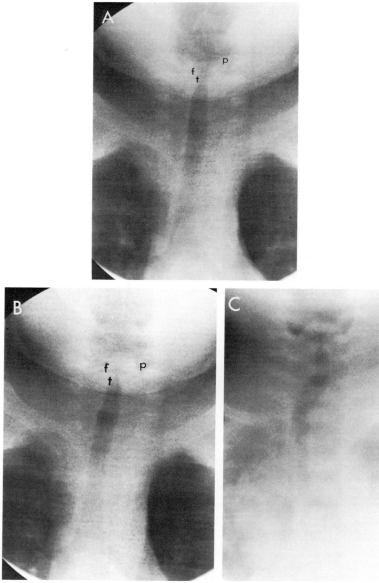

Fig 3–5.—The dynamic nature of the airway. High-kilovoltage technique views show the entire airway from the vocal cords to the carina. In this sequence of three films, note that the airway buckles to the right during expiration **(C).** This is normal. (*T,* true vocal cords; *F,* false vocal cords; *P,* pyriform sinus.)

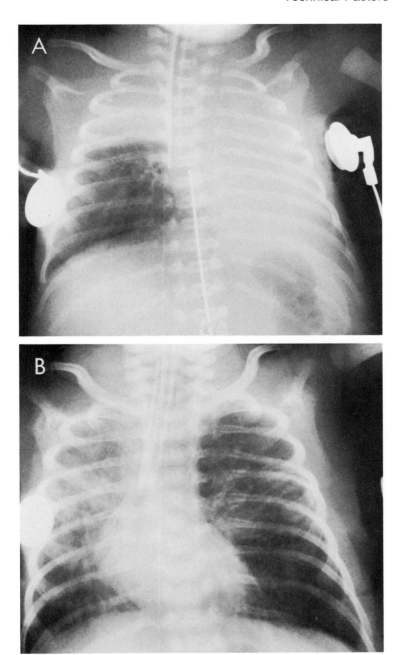

Fig 3–6.—The endotracheal tube. **A,** this is an infant with a tube in the right main-stem bronchus. Here, not only the left lung but also the right upper lobe is obstructed, as the tube is at the level of the bronchus intermedius and lower-lobe bronchus. (An umbilical arterial line is seen.) **B,** the endotracheal tube in this child is beyond the carina and acts as a ball valve, allowing the left lung to fill but not empty, causing mediastinal shift to the right. There is some atelectasis on the right. Did you see the left rib changes secondary to cardiac surgery?

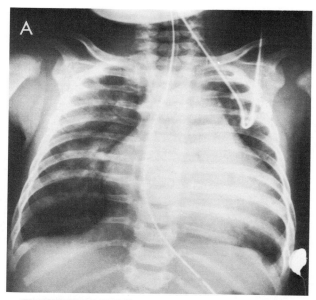

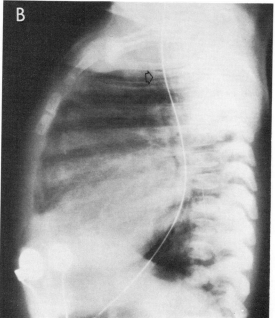

Fig 3–7.—Cardiac enlargement. **A,** frontal radiograph reveals a nasogastric tube in the stomach. The heart occupies some of the right hemithorax and extends to the left lateral hemithorax. The density behind the heart is atelectasis secondary to impingement on the left main-stem bronchus by the large heart. **B,** on the lateral film, see how the heart extends posterior to the airway, almost reaching the spine. The airway is pushed backward *(arrow).*

REED'S RULE #4—A mass must be seen in two planes, i.e., if the heart is really large, it must appear large in two planes.

If the heart is large, it should appear so in both *frontal* and *lateral views*. Since the thymus is in the anterior mediastinum, it is difficult to evaluate heart size on the frontal film. The lateral roentgenograph is most valuable in this regard (Fig 3–7). The retrocardiac air space should be seen, and when you draw a line from the anterior portion of the trachea inferiorly to the diaphragm, it should not intersect the heart (see Chap. 2).

The *contour* of the heart—the third parameter—is widely touted as being helpful in determining the specific nature of congenital heart defects. A narrow cardiac base is described in transposition of the great vessels and a "boot-shaped" heart in tetralogy of Fallot. Clinically, these signs may not be very helpful when it comes to determining an individual patient's defect, and plain-film radiography must yield to echocardiography and cardiac catheterization. However, in infants as in older children, pulmonary vascular changes may give the clue to the general category of the cardiac disease, e.g., a left-to-right shunt, etc. In contrast to the older child, the pulmonary vessels of a newborn can be seen at the hila and only in the medial third of the lungs. Vessels should be hard to find in the lateral two-thirds of the normal lung. When there is vascular plethora or increased vascularity secondary to congenital heart disease (due to a left-to-right shunt or congestive heart failure), the vascularity becomes much easier to see in the lateral two-thirds of the lung. It is much more difficult, however, to detect decreased pulmonary vascularity (as found in severe pulmonic stenosis).

DECEPTIVE SHADOWS

One of the most common mistakes that is made is diagnosing a pneumothorax when in reality it is only a skin fold (Fig 3–8). This error can be avoided by realizing

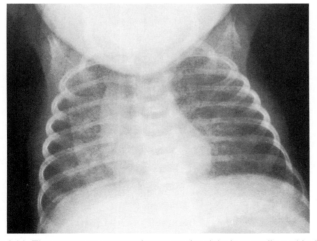

Fig 3–8.—Skin fold. The apparent pneumothorax on the right is actually a skin fold, easily determined when you realize the margin doesn't conform to the margin of the collapsed lobe or lung. If uncertain, repeat the film after moving the baby to a different position, e.g., decubitus view.

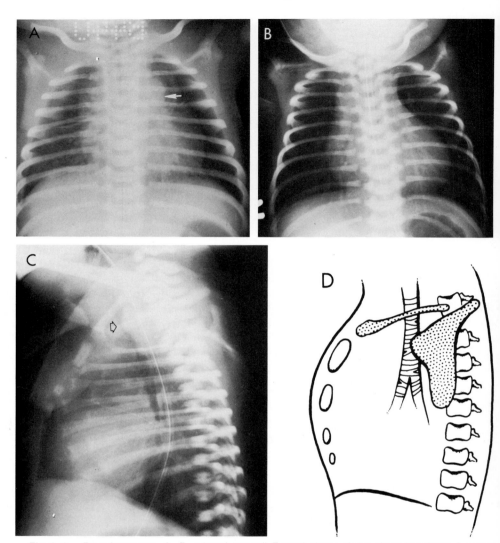

Fig 3–9.—Pseudomasses. **A, B,** "ductal bump." Frontal views of the chest in infants 1 and 3 days old, respectively. The "bump" *(arrow)* in the upper mediastinum is no longer visible. It was caused by the superimposition of the main pulmonary artery, left pulmonary artery, and ductus arteriosus. The latter gradually retracts, and the mass disappears. **C,** this lateral film shows another pseudomass. The trachea looks as if it is being compressed posteriorly by a mass *(arrow).* **D,** in fact, the "mass" is caused by superimposition of the scapula over the airway.

the border of the fold doesn't conform to the position that a collapsed lobe or lung would assume. In addition, the skin fold is frequently seen extending off into the axilla. If you are uncertain, a repeat film with the baby in another position is helpful.

Another important finding on a neonatal chest film is the "ductus bump," seen best on the frontal view at the level of the pulmonary artery (Fig 3–9). It is formed by the superimposition of the main and left pulmonary artery on the patent ductus arteriosus. It cannot be seen on the lateral film, but occasionally the scapula may mimic a pseudomass in this region.

The following summarizes the assessment of the neonatal chest and also lists questions you should be asking yourself about each film and specific parameters for evaluating the airway, mediastinal silhouette, and lungs. Remember the ABCs and Reed's Rule #1.

A. General
   1. Lung volume (Are the lungs hyperinflated?)
   2. Position of patient (Is the patient rotated? Why?)
   3. Exposure (Is the film properly exposed? How do you know?)
B. Specific
   1. Airway
      a. Patency
      b. Position
      c. Size
   2. Mediastinal silhouette
      a. Position
      b. Size
      c. Contour
   3. Lungs (see Table 3–1)
      a. Volume
      b. Pulmonary density
      c. Vascularity

AN APPROACH TO COMMON NEONATAL ABNORMALITIES

Correlation of the generalized lung volume (increased, decreased, normal) with type of pulmonary density leads to the differential diagnoses of neonatal lung disease (Table 3–1). Since the lung volume has already been assessed, differentiating

TABLE 3–1.—DIFFERENTIAL DIAGNOSIS OF LUNG PATHOLOGY BASED ON LUNG VOLUME AND TYPE OF DENSITY

LUNG VOLUME	TYPE OF DENSITY	DISEASE CONSIDERATIONS
Increased (generalized)	None	Aspiration syndromes
		Congenital heart disease
	Multiple coarse areas (strandy densities following bronchovascular pattern)	Meconium aspiration
		Retained fetal fluid
	Localized	Pneumonia
	Increased pulmonary vascularity	Congenital heart disease
Normal or decreased	Homogeneous fine granular (ground-glass) density with air bronchograms	Hyaline membrane disease
		Some form of group B β-hemolytic streptococcal pneumonia
Variable	Variable	Persistent fetal circulation; group B β-hemolytic streptotcoccal infection
Localized increase in volume	Air-filled	Lobar emphysema
	Fluid-filled	Bronchial obstruction (lobar emphysema initially, congenital cyst, bronchogenic cyst)
	Air- and/or fluid-filled	Cystic adenomatoid malformation

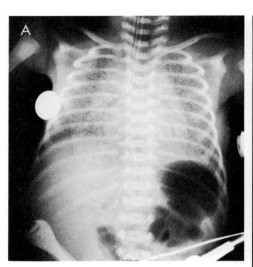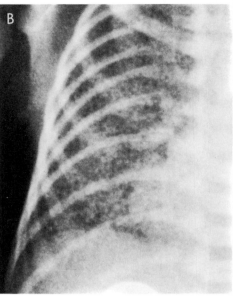

Fig 3–10.—Hyaline membrane disease. **A,** frontal radiograph of a premature infant with hyaline membrane disease demonstrates ground-glass appearance of both lungs with a normal lung volume. The endotracheal tube is in the right main-stem bronchus. **B,** frontal magnified view of the lungs with the granular appearance caused by the atelectatic surfactant-deficient alveoli.

the various forms of pulmonary density is our next task. You should ask yourself the following questions:

1. Are the densities uniform and homogeneous (Fig 3–10)?
2. Do the densities correspond to the distribution of blood vessels or bronchi (Fig 3–11)?
3. Do they involve the whole lung or a portion of the lung (Fig 3–12)?

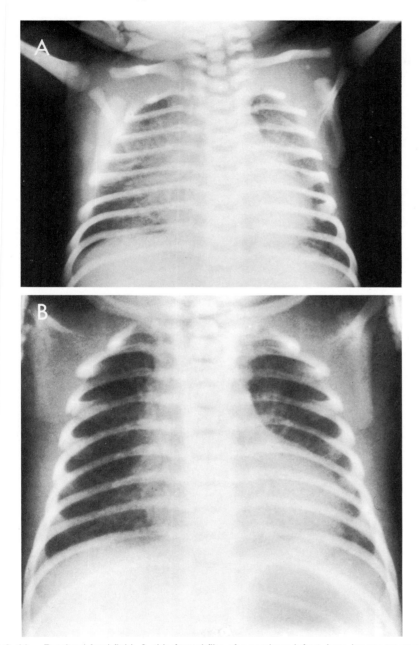

Fig 3–11.—Retained fetal fluid. **A,** this frontal film of a newborn infant, born by cesarean-section, reveals strandy densities extending from the hila throughout both lungs. The heart is not enlarged. Lung volume is mildly increased. **B,** frontal radiographs of the same child 2 days later. Chest is normal.

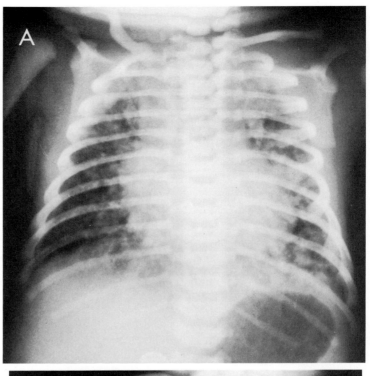

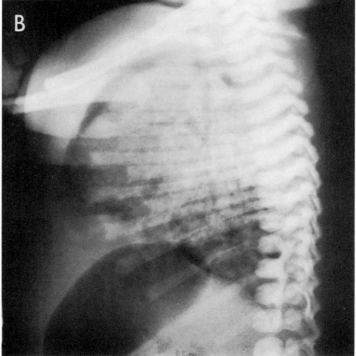

Fig 3–12.—Meconium aspiration. **A,** frontal radiograph shows coarse, globular, rounded densities dispersed throughout the lungs. Lung volume is increased. **B,** lateral view showing hyperexpansion and the coarseness throughout the lungs. The heart may be enlarged (although not in this case) in meconium aspiration secondary to anoxia.

66

DISEASES WITH GENERALIZED INCREASE IN LUNG VOLUME
(Table 3–1)

Increased lung volume may be the first and only clue to significant parenchymal or cardiovascular abnormalities in the neonate. From a teleogic point of view, the lungs are hyperexpanded as the infant tries desperately to adapt to his new environment and cannot optimally oxygenate. Any of the aspiration syndromes (discussed below), pneumonias, or congenital heart diseases may present with relatively clear lungs and hyperexpansion. However, there are frequently densities within the lung parenchyma or other clues, such as pulmonary vascularity and cardiac size (see above), that point to the correct diagnosis.

Two conditions can be readily anticipated from the changes the fetus undergoes from intrauterine to extrauterine life. First, the neonate may not be able to clear all the fetal fluid from its lungs (see Fig 3–11). Since the fluid exits through the tracheobronchial tree and is expelled when the thorax is compressed in the birth canal, tracheobronchial-tree obstruction or a cesarean section (where the baby's chest is not compressed) may lead to retained fetal fluid—the wet lung syndrome, radiographically. These babies have increased lung volume and strandy densities emanating from the hila that follow the course of the tracheobronchial tree (some bronchi, some lymphatics). Pleural fluid may be present as well; it outlines the lung fissures. While at times the retained fluid can radiographically masquerade as congestive heart failure in a neonate, the clinical picture is entirely different because babies with retained fetal fluid "pink up" easily with minimal support. Retained fetal fluid usually clears within 24–48 hours (transient tachypnea of the newborn is another name for this entity).

The second disease that can result from the birth sequence is aspiration (see Fig 3–12). The most serious kind is meconium aspiration. A fetus will pass meconium in utero because of some perinatal or parturitional stress. At the first breath, this viscous material may be inhaled. The radiograph will show increased lung

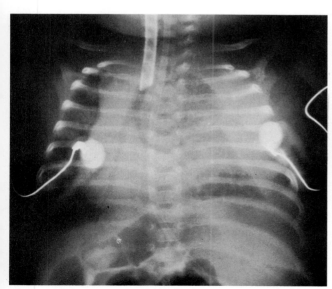

Fig 3–13.—Pneumonia. This frontal view of a 2-day-old shows extensive opacity in the left side of the chest due to both an infiltrate and a large pleural effusion. The mediastinum is shifted to the right. Beta-hemolytic streptococcus was the offending organism.

volume, but this time there are *patchy* densities through both lungs. Meconium in the tracheobronchial tree and lung parenchyma presents a striking picture (see Fig 3–12).

Early hyperexpansion of the neonatal lung may herald a localized infiltrate, such as pneumonic consolidation that does not become visible for a few days (Fig 3–13). In a neonate with congenital heart disease, the first radiographic sign may well be increased lung volume only. As pulmonary resistance decreases, signs of a left-to-right shunt or cardiac enlargement become evident. It is important to note that a large heart does not necessarily mean primary congenital heart disease; anemia, asphyxia, and other high-output states may cause cardiomegaly as well.

DISEASES WITH NORMAL OR DECREASED LUNG VOLUME (Table 3–1)

The most common disease in this group is hyaline membrane disease. Unfortunately Group B β-hemolytic streptococcal pneumonia may appear indistinguishable from it. In both diseases homogeneous, fine densities appear throughout the lungs with accompanying air bronchograms. This sign has been described as a "ground-glass appearance" (see Fig 3–10). In hyaline membrane disease, these changes are related to surfactant deficiency; therefore, the terminal air spaces tend to collapse, resulting in a low normal to decreased lung volume. The collapse of the terminal air spaces accounts for the fine, homogeneous granular densities. Remember to look for air bronchograms. You must see the granular densities or white dots all the way out to the edge of the lungs to make a diagnosis of hyaline membrane disease.

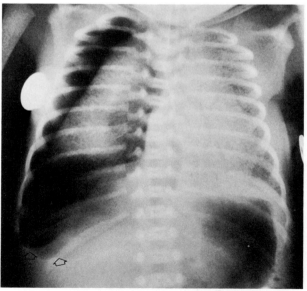

Fig 3–14.—Complications of hyaline membrane disease and ventilation. This 1-day-old infant, with hyaline membrane disease suddenly became very ill. The right lung has collapsed, and the mediastinum has shifted to the left, indicating a tension pneumothorax on the right. The large air space filling the right thoracic cavity is inverting the right hemidiaphragm *(arrows)*.

Prematurity and maternal diabetes are two of the more common underlying etiologic factors predisposing to this disease.

Mechanical ventilation often causes air to leak into the interstitium of the lungs (pulmonary interstitial emphysema), into the mediastinum (pneumomediastinum), into the pleural space (pneumothorax), and occasionally into the pericardium (pneumopericardium) (Figs 3–14 to 3–16). Rarely, air will dissect into the peritoneal cavity (Fig 3–17).

One of the most difficult conditions for the novice to recognize is the pneumomediastinum. Radiographically, there are three different densities or shades of gray visible on the frontal film (Fig 3–18). The first is the white density of the heart. The second density—the pneumomediastinum—is a radiolucent black area lateral to the heart and medial to the lungs that may elevate the thymus laterally and upward. The third is a gray density representing lung compressed laterally by trapped air.

A pneumomediastinum may be very small and may be difficult to differentiate from a pneumopericardium (see Fig 3–16). When a pneumopericardium is present, separation of the aorta from the pulmonary vein is clearly seen on both frontal and lateral views, since the pericardium attaches at the base of the great vessels. In addition, the pericardial membrane may be visible when there is air on both sides of it.

Air dissects upward into the subcutaneous tissues of the neck (unusual in a neonate) and downward through the same diaphragmatic hiatus as the aorta and esophagus, resulting in a pneumoperitoneum (see Fig 3–17).

The most important air leak, however, is that of a pneumothorax. Pneumothoraces are formed by rupture of air through the overlying pleura or by rupture of a subpleural bleb (see Fig 3–14). Once there is a rupture of air by whatever mechanism into the pleural space, the lung begins to collapse. Since the infant is recumbent, an anterior and medial air space may appear first or may outline the inferior lung margins. *Look* for the pleural margins of the lobes. Beware of skin folds that may simulate pleura (see Fig 3–8). As the quantity of air increases and the lung collapses to its fullest—i.e., the elastic limit is reached—the pressure builds up, and a *tension pneumothorax* develops. This results in:

- Shift of the mediastinum away from the midline
- Flattening or even eversion of the diaphragm on the affected side.

(If by chance the pneumothorax is bilateral, there may be no or less mediastinal shift, but then the heart is compressed and appears smaller.)

At first, these changes may be so subtle that only when compared with previous films will the tension in the pneumothorax become apparent.

> REED'S RULE #7—*Always review all old films to properly assess the new one. Subtle findings can easily be missed when a single previous examination is reviewed.*

A common problem in infants with hyaline membrane disease (HMD) is the patent ductus arteriosus (PDA), causing a left-to-right shunt. The classic roentgenographic signs of a PDA are an enlarging heart, enlarging liver, and increasing pulmonary vascularity. These, however, are late signs and may be masked by the

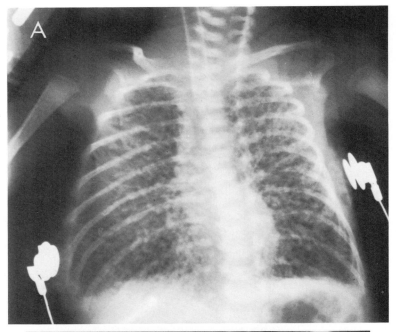

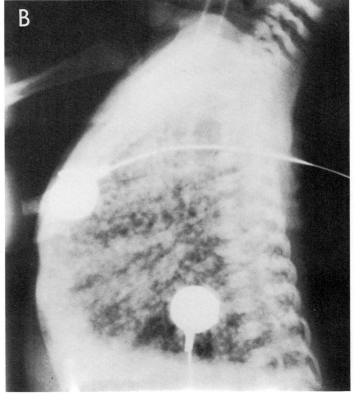

Fig 3–15.

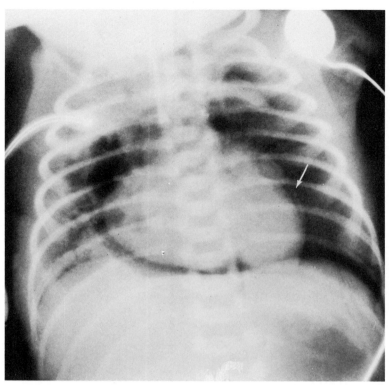

Fig 3–16.—Pneumopericardium. A frontal radiograph shows air around the heart. There is also leakage of air above the left hemidiaphragm and a pneumomediastinum. Note how the thymus is elevated by the pneumomediastinum. Arrow points to the pericardium outlined on both sides by air.

← **Fig 3–15.**—Progressive pulmonary interstitial emphysema. **A,** on this film of a 6-day-old, there is interstitial air. The high pressures necessary to ventilate the child caused air to leak into the interstitium. This may compress the bronchus and, in fact, hinder aeration. **B,** lateral view showing interstitial air as small black dots. This complication of mechanical ventilation occurs when high pressures are used and ventilation is prolonged.

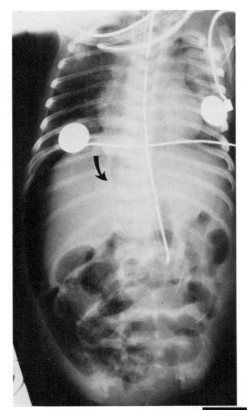

Fig 3–17.—Pneumoperitoneum. Air can dissect down the mediastinum into the peritoneal cavity. On this decubitus roentgenograph taken with the baby's right side up, free air is seen above the liver. The falciform ligament is clearly seen *(arrow).*

Fig 3–18.—Pneumomediastinum. This frontal view of the chest reveals three densities: *1,* heart; *2,* pneumomediastinum; and *3,* compressed lung.

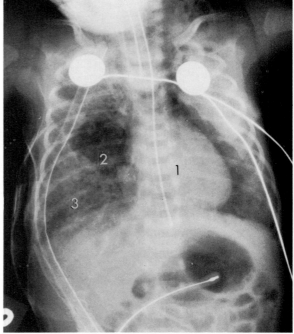

parenchymal densities of HMD. In infants with HMD, the only clues to a coexistent PDA may be (1) lack of improvement after three days of adequate therapy for HMD, and (2) increasing perihilar haze. These roentgenographic findings are frequently noted before the clinical signs of a bounding pulse or a murmur.

While most infants recover from HMD, 15%–20% go on to develop bronchopulmonary dysplasia (Fig 3–19). This disease is most likely the result of a combination of pulmonary insults due to severe hyaline membrane disease, high oxygen concentration, prematurity of the lungs, and prolonged high-pressure mechanical ventilation. Radiographically, "cystic" areas appear in the lung parenchyma, intermixed with areas of fibrosis and atelectasis (densities) and generalized emphysema. The lungs become congested secondary to "leaking" capillaries.

DISEASES WITH VARIABLE LUNG VOLUME (Table 3–1)

Persistent fetal circulation is not a radiographic diagnosis, and the neonate may present with variable lung volume.

LOCALIZED CHANGES IN LUNG VOLUME (Table 3–1)

Localized increase in lung volume can be either air-filled or fluid-filled (Fig 3–20). Since, in utero the lung is filled with fluid, an obstruction of a bronchus traps the fluid, delays resorption, and causes a localized increase in lung volume or a *"mass"* lesion. This mass compresses adjacent lobes and frequently shifts the mediastinum contralaterally. As the fluid is absorbed, it is replaced by air; but lung markings are not seen. Classically, this is associated with lobar emphysema or any condition obstructing a main-stem bronchus (e.g., intrinsic stenosis, bronchogenic cyst, pulmonary artery sling). Fine strands of tissue seen within the lucency indicate the presence of cysts. The lack of a defined *pleural* margin excludes pneumothorax.

> REED'S RULE #5—An esophagram must be done on any child with unexplained respiratory disease. It is simple, inexpensive, and informative.

In the neonate as in the older child, unexplained airway disease should prompt an esophagram, which may be done initially with a tube in the esophagus so that the "H-type" fistula between the trachea and the esophagus can be excluded (Fig 3–21). If this fistula is not found, the infant is given a bottle; and the swallowing mechanism is evaluated. Look at the position, course, contour, and motility of the esophagus. A vascular ring, i.e., an anomaly of the great vessels, often impinges on the esophagus and the airway. Masses or nodes at the carina can do this as well. Check for gastroesophageal reflux—chalasia—during this examination (see Chap. 5). In addition, under fluoroscopy, the diaphragm and mediastinum can be examined for diaphragmatic paralysis and unilateral air-trapping.

If, after this study, further airway evaluation is necessary or if the child continues to be a "noisy neonate," the airway can be studied fluoroscopically with the use of videotape and high-kilovoltage technique (see Chap. 9).

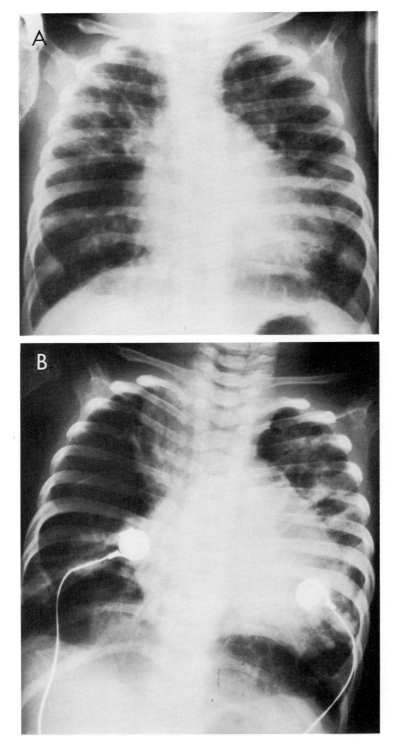

Fig 3–19.

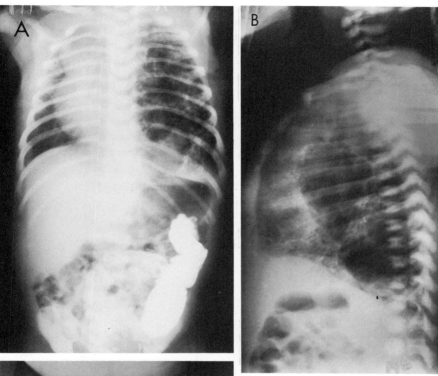

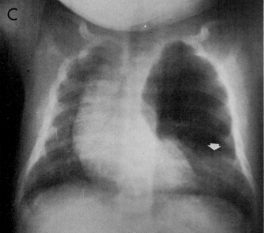

Fig 3–20.—Multiple causes of localized increase in lung volume. **A,** frontal radiograph of neonate, with shift of the mediastinum to the right and cystic changes involving most of the left hemithorax. The bowel pattern is seen in the abdomen and is normal, so the chest findings are not caused by herniation of bowel loops. **B,** on the lateral film, large cysts can be seen. This child had cystic adenomatoid malformation, a hamartoma of the lung. **C,** lobar emphysema. Note the localized increase in lung volume in the left upper lobe. The left lower lobe is compressed *(arrow)*.

← **Fig 3–19.**—Sequelae of hyaline membrane disease and mechanical ventilation. **A,** this 6-month-old had severe hyaline membrane disease requiring assisted ventilation for over 1 month; he was still on supplemental oxygen. The heart is enlarged, and there are fibrous changes throughout both lungs with uneven expansion. The lungs are very hyperexpanded. **B,** at 1 year of age, further enlargement of the heart has occurred, and there is increasing emphysema. The areas of fibrosis have now coalesced. There is some cyst formation in the left midlung and left base. This child died at 18 months of age of chronic respiratory insufficiency.

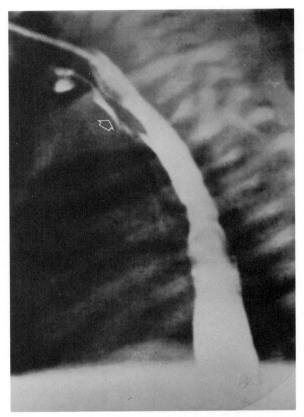

Fig 3–21.—"H-type" tracheoesophageal fistula in a child with chronic pneumonia. This lateral view of an esophagram demonstrates an unusual finding. A small barium-filled tract *(arrow)* can be seen from the esophagus running upward toward the trachea. Ingested food could similarly be aspirated into the lungs.

Remember, the most important question is, "Why am I ordering this set of films?". Once the diagnosis of hyaline membrane disease or severe bronchopulmonary dysplasia is established, radiographs should be used to show correctable conditions, such as airway obstruction, pneumonia, pneumothoraces, vascular rings, etc. Since the premature infant may be more acutely sensitive to the deleterious effects of radiation (Chap. 1), the timing and selection of radiographic examinations should be tempered with this consideration.

SUGGESTED READING

1. Swischuk L.E.: *Radiology of the Newborn and Young Infant*, ed. 2. Baltimore, Williams & Wilkins Co., 1980.
2. Caffey J.: *Pediatric X-ray Diagnosis*, ed. 7. Chicago, Year Book Medical Publishers, Inc., 1978.

CHAPTER 4

The Gastrointestinal Tract

ROENTGENOGRAPHIC INTERPRETATION of a child's abdomen is a challenging experience, as there are many subtle clues to the nature of the disease process. Appropriate interpretation requires both knowledge of the technical aspects of how the film was made and a systematic approach.

TECHNICAL FACTORS

In the discussion of the chest, you learned that observing gravitational effects is useful in assessing a film. This is also true in the abdomen: i.e., air always rises; fluid goes to the dependent area.

>*REED'S RULE #8—The abdominal examination should include a minimum of three views—supine, prone, and erect.*

Think of the air in the abdomen as contrast medium; the purpose of obtaining three views is to move air into different loops of bowel so that the maximal quantity of bowel can be visualized. With the patient supine, what portions of the bowel are highest? The answer, of course, is the transverse colon and the body of the stomach. Therefore, on the abdominal supine film, air rises to these regions (Fig 4–1). When the patient is prone, the highest portions of the bowel are the ascending and descending colon, the rectum, and the fundus of the stomach. Therefore, gas should rise to these areas (see Fig 4–1). Remembering these facts can frequently help you to distinguish large from small bowel. Look carefully at the bones on the supine film. The iliac wings appear larger and more rounded than they do on the prone film (see Fig 4–1).

The erect view is the last film in the series. (Decubitus will do if the patient is too sick or unable to stand.) How do you know if the film is an erect view? Once again, remember the effects of gravity. There is an air-fluid level in the stomach. Similarly, if the bowel contains fluid, you will see multiple air-fluid levels. Notice how most of the bowel falls into the lower abdomen and pelvis, while the gastric fundus remains fixed in the left upper quadrant. You can see the colon in the flanks, with the transverse segment extending from beneath the liver, across the abdomen below the stomach into the left upper quadrant.

THE RADIOLOGIST'S CIRCLE AND THE ABC'S

In a child with acute abdominal distress, it is not uncommon to take sequential examinations of the abdomen. Therefore, it is important to check the date and time of examination in the corner of the film. Progressing in our imaginary circle, the

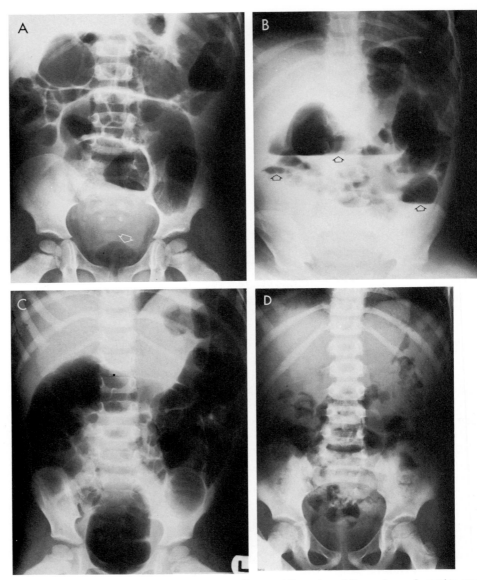

Fig 4–1.—The value of air as a contrast medium and the value of three views. **A,** supine roentgenograph in this 18-month-old with abdominal pain reveals multiple loops of bowel in the midabdomen but little gas within the rectum *(arrow)*. On this film, you are not sure if the air is in the large or the small bowel. **B,** an erect film reveals multiple air-fluid levels (horizontal straight lines) *(arrows)* throughout the abdomen. The base of the lungs is clear. **C,** prone examination reveals gas in the rectum and the sigmoid, ascending, and descending colon. The predominant pattern is that of colonic gas. The small bowel is not distended, and there is no evidence of obstruction. **D,** normal abdomen. Evaluate it systematically.

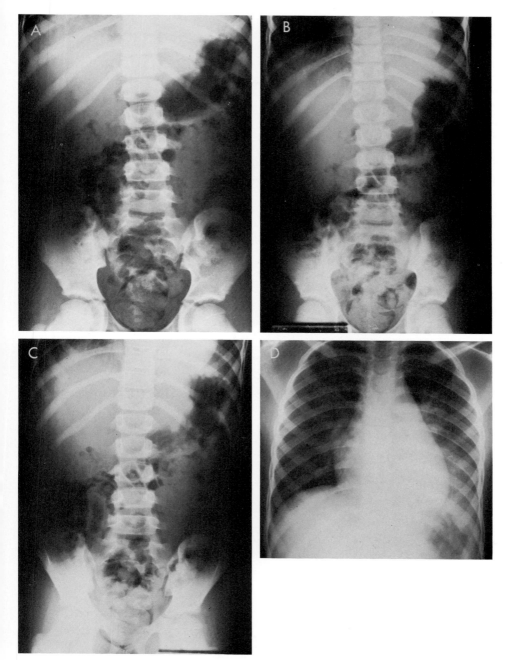

Fig 4–2.—On every abdominal film, examine the chest as if you were actually reading a chest film. **A,** supine view of the abdomen reveals a normal bowel gas pattern; but there is a suggestion of a density behind the left side of the heart, and the left diaphragm is not visible. **B,** on the erect film, notice how most of the bowel falls inferiorly into the lower abdomen, while the gastric fundus is fixed and filled with air. Above and medial to the gastric fundus, the left lung density and "silhouetted" diaphragm are again noted. **C,** on the prone film, gas moves to the flanks. Note the left lung base. **D,** the chest examination reveals pneumonia in the left lower lobe; the left side of the diaphragm is not visible. You must remember to look through the liver density on the right and the gastric air bubble on the left to see basilar infiltrates on any abdominal series.

ABCs should be reviewed, but this time in the reverse order: *chest, bones and soft tissues,* and (in this instance) *abdomen.*

> *REED'S RULE #9—On every abdominal examination, evaluate the chest as if you were looking at a chest film.*

CHEST

It is often easier to see basilar lung changes, fractures of the lower ribs and pleural reactions on an abdominal film than on a chest film (Fig 4–2). In addition, the chest film may not adequately show a low thoracic paraspinal mass, which is readily spotted on abdominal films. Remember, the posterior lung sulcus is located at the level of the 12th thoracic vertebra. To find it, you must look *through* the liver density on the right and the gastric air bubble on the left.

BONES AND SOFT TISSUES

The bones and soft tissues can provide extremely valuable information. In making our imaginary radiologist's circle, note whether there is swelling or edema of the soft tissues, as represented by a nonhomogeneous pattern. It is also important to

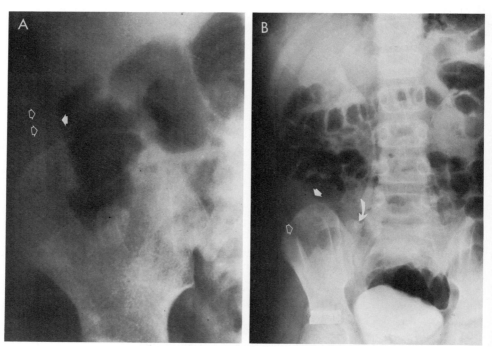

Fig 4–3.—Properitoneal fat line. **A,** close-up view of the right lower quadrant shows the dark, linear properitoneal fat line *(open arrows),* with the descending colon only a few millimeters away *(solid arrow).* Note the appendicolith. At this time, the child was asymptomatic. **B,** 1 month later, the child became febrile and suffered right lower quadrant pain. Intravenous urogram shows the bowel *(solid straight arrow)* now displaced from the properitoneal fat line *(open arrow).* The appendicolith *(curved arrow)* is also displaced. A large appendiceal abscess was discovered at surgery.

identify the properitoneal fat line (Fig 4–3). This radiolucent line is the lateral margin of the peritoneal cavity; the gas-filled ascending colon and frequently the descending colon are within 1–2 mm of this line on the prone film. A separation between the properitoneal fat line and the colon on the prone film indicates the presence of fluid or possibly an intra-abdominal mass. Remember, this sign is only useful if the colon has air in it (see Fig 4–3)!

The lower ribs, spine, and pelvis are the major bones of concern on the abdominal film. Since specific abnormalities of these bones will be discussed in Chapter 7, the major item of concern now is symmetry. Asymmetry must always be explained. Once again, abnormalities of bone should lead to careful searching of neighboring intra-abdominal contents; i.e., left lower rib fractures should make you suspect renal or splenic injury.

ABDOMEN

In the systematic approach, we look last at the area for which the film was requested. Therefore, our approach to the intra-abdominal contents is to view the muscles, soft tissues, and viscera before examining the bowel gas pattern. Begin at the top of the film, most often with the erect film, looking for signs of free intraperitoneal air. As you can see in Figure 4–1,B, the diaphragm on the left is easily visible because of the stomach bubble. On the right, the liver is directly beneath the diaphragm; and only the top margin—the thoracic margin—can be seen. Since air rises on the erect film, free air collects between the liver and diaphragm on the right and between the stomach bubble and the diaphragm on the left. On the supine film, however, air rises and fills the space above the viscera and beneath the umbilicus and the abdominal musculature. Free air is more difficult to see on this view but should nevertheless be recognized, as there is a subtle change in the soft tissue density of the abdomen (Fig 4–4). The liver may be less dense (blacker) than the soft tissues. Therefore, there will be three densities, proceeding from the lateral aspect of the right side: (1) the soft tissue density; (2) the liver density, which is somewhat darker; and (3) the stomach density full of air, which is the darkest. Normally, there are only two densities—the liver and soft tissues (which are of equal density) and the air in the stomach.

The falciform ligament is never normally visible; it can only be seen when surrounded by free intraperitoneal air. This ligament courses downward from its diaphragmatic attachment between the margin of the right and left lobes of the liver to the lowest aspect of the umbilical remnants. When there is free intraperitoneal air, the large bubble of free air assumes an oval configuration with the falciform ligament being central—the laces of a football—in the football sign (see Fig 4–4).

Continuing with your appraisal of the film from the top down, look at the liver and spleen and assess their size, if possible (see Fig 4–1, D). A radiologist measures liver size only infrequently; hepatic enlargement is usually an impression. The spleen is often obscured by bowel gas. Remember, a good inspiration will push the liver down, while a poor inspiration will, in fact, let the liver rise.

Determination of splenic size and position is usually possible by locating the inferior and medial margins. The stomach air bubble and gas in the splenic flexure of the colon lie immediately adjacent to the spleen; and both may be displaced, particularly if the spleen is enlarged. Inasmuch as one can feel beneath the costal

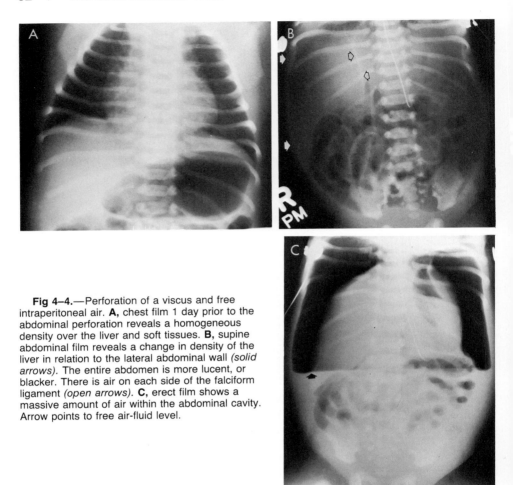

Fig 4–4.—Perforation of a viscus and free intraperitoneal air. **A,** chest film 1 day prior to the abdominal perforation reveals a homogeneous density over the liver and soft tissues. **B,** supine abdominal film reveals a change in density of the liver in relation to the lateral abdominal wall *(solid arrows)*. The entire abdomen is more lucent, or blacker. There is air on each side of the falciform ligament *(open arrows)*. **C,** erect film shows a massive amount of air within the abdominal cavity. Arrow points to free air-fluid level.

margin to palpate a spleen, reference of the splenic density to this margin helps you decide whether or not it is actually enlarged. Ask yourself, "Could I palpate it?" If so, "How big did it feel?"

Proceeding inferiorly on the film, note the iliopsoas muscles attached to the spine at the upper lumbar vertebra and proceed diagonally and laterally to the lesser trochanters of the femora. The lateral margins can usually be seen. The key to identifying pathology of the psoas margins is asymmetry. If a portion of the psoas muscle is not visible while the rest of the muscle and the opposite one are, abnormal soft-tissue densities in this region should be considered. The entire psoas margins sometimes cannot be seen on films of infants and children with abundant fecal material or bowel gas (see Fig 4–1, *D*).

The kidneys are adjacent to the lateral margin of the iliopsoas muscles. More will be said about them in Chapter 5.

Look specifically for calcifications in all areas of the abdomen. Stones in the gallbladder, urinary tract, pancreas, or appendix are prone to occur if there is stasis or an inflammation (Fig 4–5). Benign and malignant neoplasms can calcify. Once a calcification has been identified and anatomically located, characterize it. Is it sharply marginated and of uniform density? Is it laminated? (This indicates it has been there for a long time, and the chemical processes have varied so different layers are formed.) Is it well formed and flocculent, as found in adrenal calcifications; or is it punctate with poorly defined margins, representing irregular deposition in a necrotic, rapidly growing neoplastic process? What is the calcification doing to the system in which it resides? Is it producing obstruction, or is it ulcerating? Does it look "physiologic"? A phlebolith in an infant is definitely abnormal but may be "normal" in an adult. The same situation is true for vascular (tubular) calcifications (see Figs 4–3 and 4–5).

Continuing downward on the three views of the abdomen, evaluate the soft tissues of the pelvis for asymmetry. The bladder appears as a smooth and round soft tissue mass when distended. In infants, it tends to extend up into the right lower quadrant.

Finally, look at the bowel-gas pattern. Figure 4–2 shows a normal bowel gas pattern in an older child, while Figure 4–6 shows a normal bowel gas pattern in a neonate. Even though there is a large amount of gas in the neonatal abdomen, the bowel loops have a recognizable, polygonal pattern. In neonates with bowel distention, the loops become "sausage-shaped"; it is frequently impossible to tell large from small bowel, but even here, the three views will help.

Observe the bowel-gas pattern for *position, contour,* and *size* (distention). The bowel may be displaced by a mass (Fig 4–7, see also Chap. 6). When you compare Figures 4–2, 4–6, and 4–7, the presence of a soft tissue mass is striking. Free intraperitoneal fluid causes the bowel to move centrally and imparts a gray or hazy appearance to the abdomen (Fig 4–8). The sharp liver angle (margin) is obscured by the fluid. Any fluid, be it lymph, blood, pus, etc., can give this appearance. Here again, however, we can use the effects of gravity to our advantage. Air in the bowel will float centrally, with the fluid in the dependent portions (see Fig 4–8).

The contour of the bowel is discussed under "Contrast Examinations" (pp. 88–89). However, we use air as much as possible because it is a good contrast agent. The bowel margins should be smooth, not ragged or irregular. The contour should change as position changes, implying pliability; it should not be rigid. If a space-occupying lesion—a mass—pushes on adjacent segments of bowel and changes the contour, the wall appears stretched as a result of the extrinsic pressure.

An increase in the size and amount of bowel distention is crucial to the diagnosis of intra-abdominal disease. Children normally have some small-bowel gas or (on the erect film) even an occasional air-fluid level in the colon. While *multiple* small bowel and colonic fluid levels are seen in mechanical bowel obstruction, they are also seen in infants as well as older children *without* obstructive bowel disease. Many of these children will have nothing more threatening than gastroenteritis (see Fig 4–1). However, if you cannot see air in the colon or rectum, or if there is a *localized* distention of bowel, you should be very suspicious of underlying pathologic changes. In crying children, the stomach may be quite large without any pathology. However, localized distention of small bowel provides a valuable clue to the site of disease—a *sentinel loop* (Fig 4–9). Remember:

REED'S RULE #2—Knowledge of anatomy is the key to correct radio-graphic diagnosis.

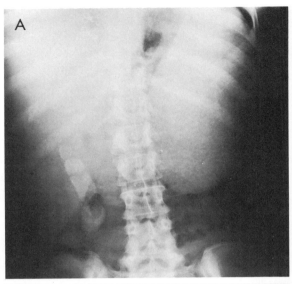

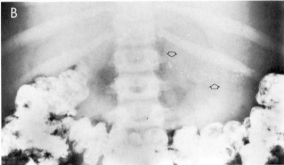

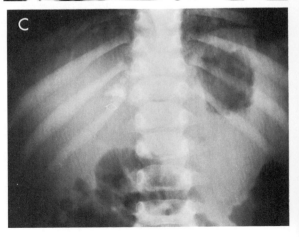

Fig 4–5.—Calcifications within the abdomen. **A,** 16-year-old with several areas of calcification. The first is a tubular density in the right midabdomen. This is a gallbladder which contained multiple radiopaque gallstones. The second is a large viscus in the left upper quadrant with punctate calcifications representing an enlarged spleen, which has undergone iron replacement secondary to multiple transfusions for hemolytic anemia (hemochromatosis). **B,** this 15-year-old with cystic fibrosis and diabetes mellitus has calcifications in the region of the pancreas. A coned-down view from the barium enema shows that they extend the entire length, from the head to the tail, of the pancreas *(arrows)*. **C,** 6½-year-old child examined for urinary tract infection. At the 12th right rib there are coarse, triangular calcifications *(arrow),* which appear in the vicinity of the adrenal gland and are the end result of neonatal adrenal hemorrhage.

What viscera are these sentinel loops near? What vessels are found in this area? What type of pathology commonly occurs in this quadrant?

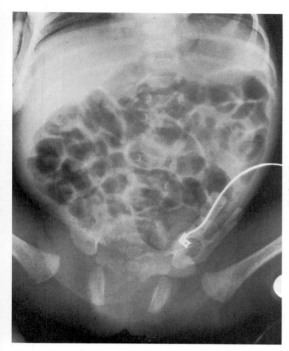

Fig 4–6.—Normal bowel pattern in a neonate. This abdominal film shows bowel loops that display a polygonal pattern. On this particular film, gas is not seen in the rectum.

Fig 4–7.—Abnormal gas pattern. A supine film of a 4-year-old with a protruberant abdomen reveals a large, homogeneous density over the right and midabdomen. The bowel gas is pushed to the left. A sonographic examination confirmed the presence of a mesenteric cyst.

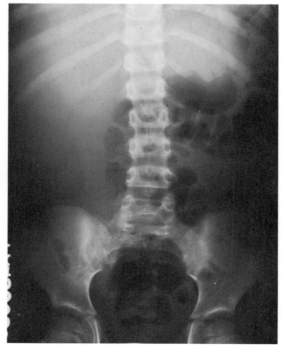

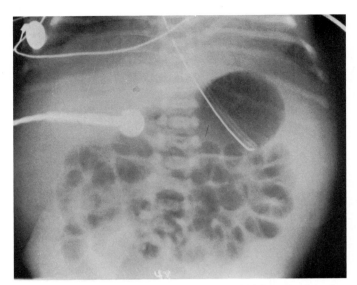

Fig 4–8.—Ascites. On this supine radiograph of a 2-day-old infant, the bowel gas is pushed to the center, and there is a grayness to the flanks. The fluid moved appropriately on multiple views because it was free ascitic fluid, secondary to urinary obstruction and posterior urethral valves. Note how the bowel loops float centrally instead of being displaced to one side by a mass, as in Figure 4–7.

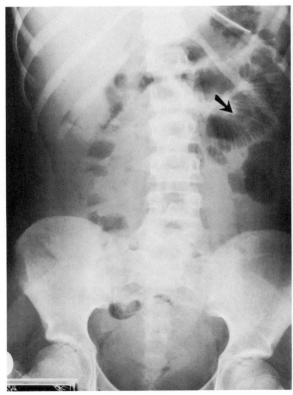

Fig 4–9.—Sentinel loop. There is a localized distention of small bowel in the left upper quadrant *(arrow)*. It is clearly identifiable as small bowel because of the valvulae conniventes (Parallel lines). The sentinel loop remained in this region on multiple views. The child had blunt abdominal trauma, and the sentinel loop was anterior to an inflamed pancreas.

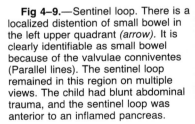

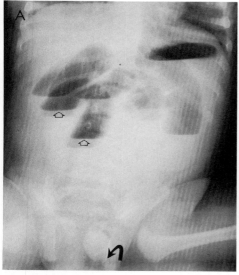

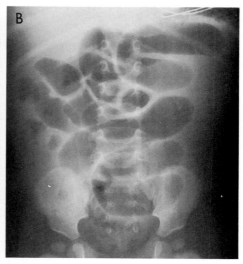

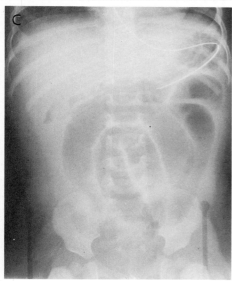

Fig 4–10.—Small bowel obstruction. This 1-year-old had an incarcerated inguinal hernia. **A,** erect film shows multiple air-fluid levels. Small bowel loop's interface at different levels (stepladder appearance [*arrows*]) may be helpful in differentiating between obstruction and absence of peristalsis. Note the air in the groin *(curved arrow).* **B,** supine radiograph shows large, distended loops in a stepladder pattern in the midabdomen. **C,** on prone film, gas has not successfully shifted into the colon. The largest loops remain in the midabdomen. Small-bowel obstruction is present.

Increase in bowel size (distention) may occur in both small and large bowel without obstruction, but there is a *recognizable pattern to the distention.* The small bowel is less distended than the colon, and there is gas in the rectum. This condition has been called paralytic (without peristalsis) ileus (distention). Figure 4–1 is such an example, and this child has gastroenteritis. However, patients who have been given atropine derivatives or who have dysmotility syndrome may have the same radiographic picture. Since the patient with gastroenteritis will have normal to increased peristalsis and the patient given atropine derivatives will have decreased peristalsis, the term *ileus* is somewhat confusing. It is best to describe the pattern and allow the clinician to fit it into the patient's status.

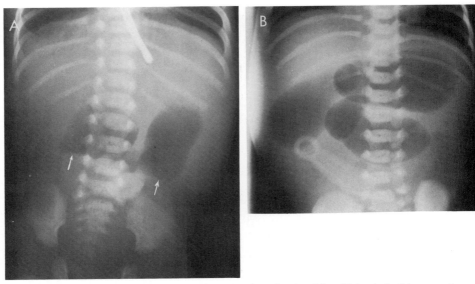

Fig 4–11.—Mechanical bowel obstruction at various levels of the GI tract. **A,** this neonate presented with vomiting. The radiographs of the abdomen reveal two air-fluid levels *(arrows)* one in the stomach and one in the duodenum. This child had duodenal atresia. **B,** this 1-day-old presented abruptly with vomiting after feeding. Supine abdominal film reveals three air-containing structures—the stomach, duodenum, and jejunum. At surgery, this child was found to have jejunal atresia.

A *more uniform,* generalized increase of all or parts of the small or large bowel along with multiple air-fluid levels and no air in the rectum denotes mechanical bowel obstruction (Fig 4–10). The site of obstruction is determined by how much bowel is distended. That is, many loops mean distal bowel obstruction, while a few distended loops mean proximal bowel obstruction (Fig 4–11). The curvature or contour of the loops of distended bowel is acute—hairpin turns—and the fluid levels are uneven, i.e., a stepladder distribution. Because of the hyperperistalsis, the bowel beyond the obstruction is devoid of gas (assuming the process has been present for some time).

ROUTINE CONTRAST EXAMINATIONS

Barium sulfate is used to coat the *intraluminal surface* of the bowel in order to reveal mucosal, submucosal, and extrinsic masses impinging on or constricting the lumen. By filling the bowel under fluoroscopic control, the radiologist can observe distensibility, pliability, and intraluminal content. Peristaltic activity, particularly in the upper gastrointestinal tract, is also carefully observed. These features are important when one suspects neoplasm or inflammation. The intricacies of these radiologic examinations are beyond the scope of this text. In general, the patient is placed in multiple positions while barium is introduced either orally or rectally under direct vision, i.e., fluoroscopic control. Films are obtained with the patient in many positions so that air and barium coat different portions of the bowel.

THE ESOPHAGUS

Evaluation of the upper gastrointestinal tract begins with an esophagram, (Fig 4–12) and some of the indications for this procedure are discussed in Chapter 2.

REED'S RULE #5—An esophagram must be done on any child with unexplained respiratory disease.

Many abnormalities of the esophagus (foreign body, duplication, etc.) and disorders of the swallowing mechanism may lead to respiratory distress secondary to aspiration and/or compression of the airway. On an esophagram, the entire nasopharynx, oropharynx, and hypopharynx, as well as the esophagus, from its origin at the inferior margin of the pyriform sinuses to the diaphragm, should be seen (see Fig 4–12). It is important to see that the nasopharynx is not filled with contrast, as this manifestation of swallowing dysfunction can cause choking and aspiration. As with all examinations, it is crucial to look at adjacent structures, i.e., the airway, to make sure there is no compression, displacement, or contrast material within the trachea. It is important to study the esophagus for *position, contour,* and *size.* The fluoroscopist evaluates the motility of the esophagus, but this is difficult to ascertain on plain films alone.

In evaluating the *position* of the esophagus, note that, in the lateral projection, there should be no separation between the anterior wall of the esophagus and the posterior wall of the trachea. On frontal examinations, the esophagus overlies the right side of the spine, passing through the intrathoracic portion until it crosses the spine distally. The esophagogastric junction is to the left of the spine.

The *contours* of the esophagus are smooth, with specific, normal indentations (see Fig 4–12). The first is the cricopharyngeal muscle, a smooth posterior indentation in the cervical region at the C-5 level.

REED'S RULE #10—In obstruction of a lumen, there should be proximal distention.

It is unusual for the cricopharyngeal muscle to cause a problem, except in severe neurologic impairment. The next two indentations on the barium column are seen on the frontal radiograph: the first at the level of the aortic arch and the next at the level of the left main-stem bronchus. Foreign bodies, when ingested, usually are found in these regions (see Fig 4–13), as are vascular anomalies.

The *size* of the esophagus changes with peristalsis. The fluoroscopist sees a wave beginning above and proceeding uniformly through the esophagus until it empties its contents into the stomach. This is a stripping wave. Conditions with abnormal motility are usually detected at this time. On any single film, one area of the esophagus may be more dilated or constricted than another, but this should be a transitory phenomenon. A specific area of normal intermittent widening is in the distal one-third of the esophagus, just above the gastroesophageal junction. This is a good place to detect esophageal varices or hiatal hernia.

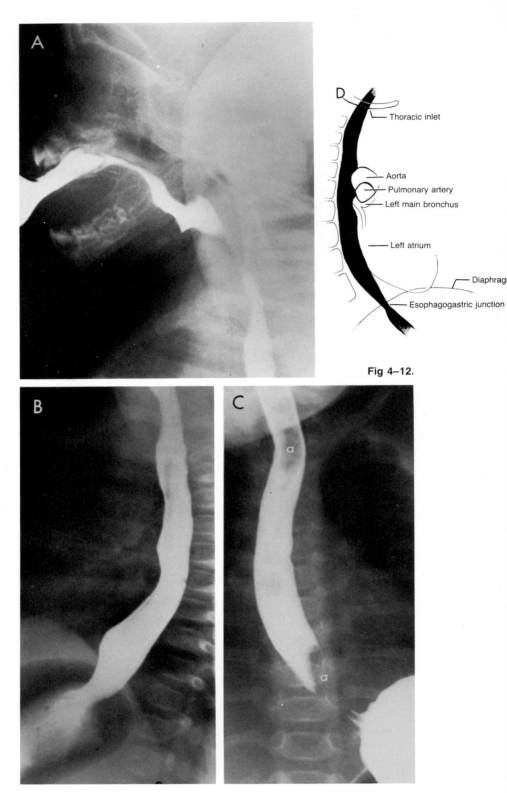

Fig 4–12.

Thoracic inlet

Aorta

Pulmonary artery

Left main bronchus

Left atrium

Diaphragm

Esophagogastric junction

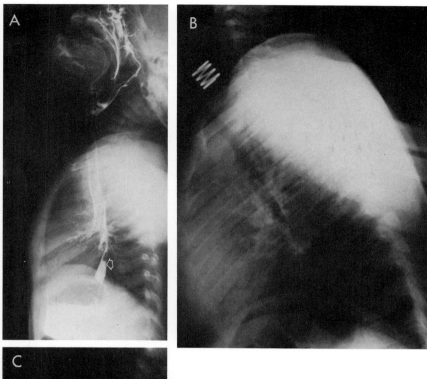

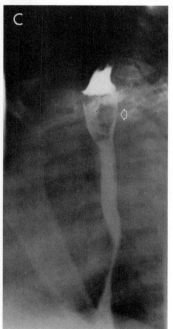

Fig 4–13.—Esophageal abnormalities. **A,** this infant has swallowing difficulty and nasal reflux. It choked and aspirated the contrast, which is now seen in the esophagus posteriorly *(arrow)* and in the tracheobronchial tree anteriorly. **B,** this 16-month-old had a radiopaque spring in the esophagus. The cricopharyngeus muscle at the thoracic inlet is one of the areas of physiologic narrowing. Frequently, children with esophageal foreign bodies can present with airway symptoms due to impingement entirely on the trachea. **C,** the aortic arch is another site of physiologic narrowing. When this food substance *(arrow)* was removed, no stricture was found. If a foreign body is stuck at an area other than a normal site of narrowing, a stricture should be suspected.

← **Fig 4–12.**—The normal esophagram. **A,** films are taken routinely in the frontal and lateral projections. In this lateral view, the swallowing mechanism is observed, and the contrast is noted in the oropharynx, hypopharynx, and proximal esophagus. There is no nasal reflux. Barium in the nasopharynx indicates swallowing dysfunction. **B,** the entire esophagus is visualized, as well as the esophagogastric junction. The walls are smooth and undulate gently. There are no mass impressions upon the esophagus. **C,** frontal view reveals a distended esophagus and some air bubbles in the esophagus. *(a)*. **D,** drawing of the lateral view of the barium-filled esophagus with the *physiologic* areas of narrowing.

THE UPPER GASTROINTESTINAL SERIES

The upper GI series (Fig 4–14) includes visualization of the esophagus, as well as the stomach, duodenum, and ligament of Treitz. This ligament is the fibrous

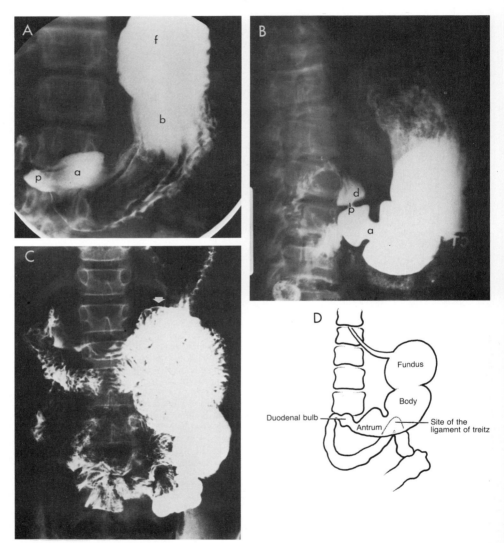

Fig 4–14.—The upper gastrointestinal series. **A,** the stomach is visualized in multiple positions so that contrast is moved through the fundus *(f)*, body *(b)*, antrum *(a)*, and pyloric region *(p)*. The mucosal pattern is smooth and regular without any disruptions. Peristaltic waves can be deduced by the various shapes of the stomach, noted on multiple films as well as at fluoroscopy. **B,** oblique view shows to advantage the contraction at the antrum *(a)* and the pyloric channel *(p)*. The duodenal bulb *(d)* is triangular and smooth. The duodenum is partially filled. **C,** further along in the study, the duodenum is entirely filled, and the ligament of Treitz *(arrow)*, behind the stomach, is at the level of the duodenal bulb. The jejunal pattern appears feathery and unobstructed. **D,** drawing of the proximal stomach to the jejunum.

band that fixes the duodenal-jejunal junction to the posterior peritoneal wall on the left of the spine at a cephalic height equal to that of the duodenal bulb. The upper GI examination is useful for detecting ulcers or masses within the stomach, ulcers or obstruction of the duodenum, and malrotation, a condition in which the duodenal-jejunal junction is not properly affixed by the ligament of Treitz. Failure of this fixation often results in obstruction of the duodenum, either by peritoneal bands or twisting of the duodenum and subsequent midgut volvulus. An upper GI series can also detect masses within the epigastrium that may impinge on the duodenal sweep, as well as inflammatory bowel disease of the duodenum. Congenital anomalies of the stomach and duodenum can be seen. Direct visualization of the liver, gallbladder, and pancreas cannot be obtained by this method.

The stomach is then studied in its entirety by placing the patient in various positions and using the effects of gravity to move the liquid barium and air content from one area to another. The mucosal pattern is formed by the gastric rugae throughout the fundus, body, and antrum of the stomach. The *contours* of the stomach are smooth, and the stomach narrows in an expected manner at the pyloric channel (there is also intermittent contraction at the antrum). The pyloric channel is 1–3 mm long and readily opens into the duodenal bulb (see Fig 4–14). It is important to recognize the normal pyloric channel, as this is the site of pyloric stenosis in young infants.

The duodenum is divided into four parts: the bulb, the vertical portion, the transverse portion, and the ascending portion (see Fig 4–14). The vertical and transverse portions form the C loop and are the retroperitoneal portions of the duodenum. The medial margin of the duodenum is adjacent to the head of the pancreas, while the lateral margin is adjacent to the liver and gallbladder. It is important to note the *contours* and *position* of the duodenum, as masses or abnormalities in adjacent structures will affect the duodenum and cause distortion. It is also important to view the duodenum in frontal and lateral projections to detect anterior or posterior deviation. The transverse portion of the duodenum crosses the spine from right to left, and the ascending portion ends at the ligament of Treitz to the left of the spine and assumes a position at the height of the duodenal bulb (see Fig 4–13).

SMALL BOWEL FOLLOW-THROUGH

This study (Fig 4–15) includes visualization of the esophagus, upper GI tract, and small bowel to the ileocecal valve. It is the examination of choice in children with suspected inflammatory bowel disease such as Crohn's disease. The study is also useful in defining partial distal small-bowel obstruction. Immediately beyond the ligament of Treitz, jejunum begins in the left upper quadrant and runs from left to right. The jejunal-ileal junction is *not* a clearly defined landmark. The mucosal pattern of the small bowel has been described as feathery. This is caused by the valvulae conniventes—Kerckring's folds. In contrast to the colon, these are transverse, circular muscles that convolute the mucosa (see Fig 4–15).

The terminal ileum has a nodular appearance in children due to the lymphoid tissue of Peyer's patches. This is normal and not, as in an adult, associated with an immune-deficient state.

In a small-bowel series, it is important that all loops be filled at some point, and

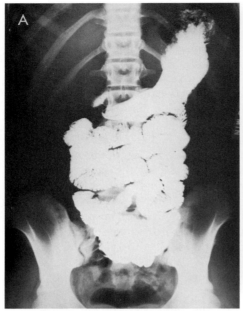

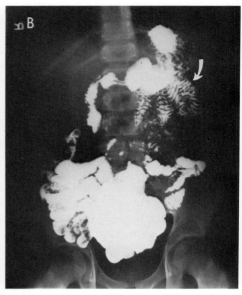

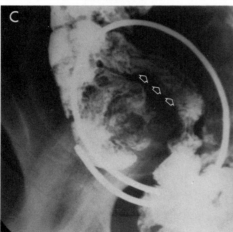

Fig 4–15.—Small-bowel follow-through. **A,** a film taken 30 minutes after the upper portion of the gastrointestinal tract was viewed reveals that the proximal half of the small bowel is now filled. The demarcation between the jejunum and ileum is difficult to see, but bowel is filling on both the right and left sides of the midline. The loops are not significantly separated. **B,** 2-hour film shows that contrast has advanced into the proximal colon; the feathery pattern of the jejunum is still visible *(arrow)*. **C,** the terminal ileum *(arrows)* is best demonstrated by compressing it with a balloon paddle and taking a spot film. This method helps evaluate the cecum, ileocecal valve, and terminal ileum.

adjacent loops should not appear unduly separated when filled. The feathery mucosal pattern of the valvulae should have no irregularity or ulceration. Once the barium is swallowed, it takes 30 minutes to 2 hours to reach the ileocecal valve in most children. This is variable, depending on the rate of gastric emptying.

BARIUM ENEMA

In this study (Fig 4–16), contrast is introduced through the rectum until the entire colon is filled. By coating the intraluminal surfaces of the colon, polyps, diverticula, as well as ulcerations and fistulous tracts, inflammatory bowel disease, ulcerative colitis, or Crohn's disease can be diagnosed. Masses, both intraluminal and extra-luminal, may be detected.

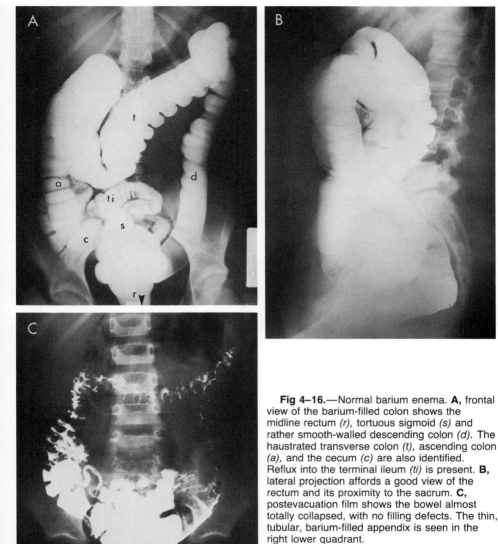

Fig 4–16.—Normal barium enema. **A,** frontal view of the barium-filled colon shows the midline rectum *(r),* tortuous sigmoid *(s)* and rather smooth-walled descending colon *(d).* The haustrated transverse colon *(t),* ascending colon *(a),* and the cecum *(c)* are also identified. Reflux into the terminal ileum *(ti)* is present. **B,** lateral projection affords a good view of the rectum and its proximity to the sacrum. **C,** postevacuation film shows the bowel almost totally collapsed, with no filling defects. The thin, tubular, barium-filled appendix is seen in the right lower quadrant.

Let's begin then with the barium enema and go through the regular film-viewing pattern. The emphasis is on the normal and the method of looking at the examination. As with other films, use the parameters of *position, contour,* and *size* when evaluating the colon. You can note the *position* of the rectum and sigmoid on the filled films. The rectum is in the midline on the frontal view, and the posterior wall lies immediately adjacent to the inner curve of the sacrum on the lateral view (see Fig 4–16). The sigmoid colon extends into the right lower quadrant and then swings

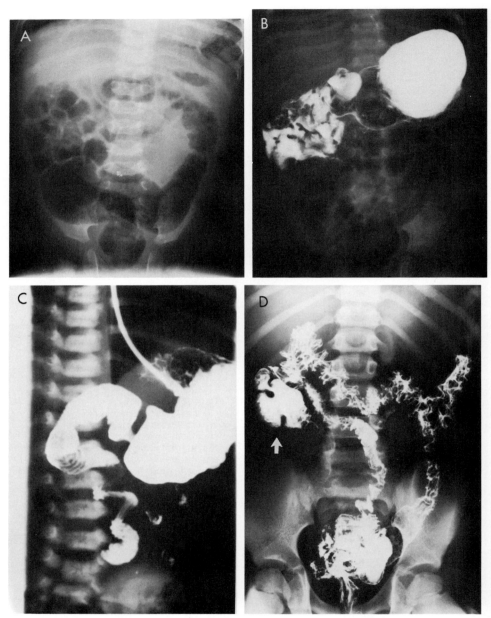

Fig 4–17.—Malrotation of midgut. **A,** plain film of the abdomen in this 5-year-old, who had been vomiting, reveals a cluster of small bowel to the right of the spine. **B,** a later film, after barium was given by mouth, shows the jejunum entirely to the right of the abdomen. The ligament of Treitz is absent. (See Fig 4–13d). **C,** spot film of the duodenum shows that the barium never goes to the normal location of the ligament of Treitz but forms a "corkscrew" pattern around the superior mesenteric artery (which is not visualized), typical of malrotation. If the duodenum gets twisted, volvulus and ischemia will result. **D,** An evacuation film following a barium enema in another patient reveals the cecum high in the right upper quadrant *(arrows)*. This is another sign of malrotation.

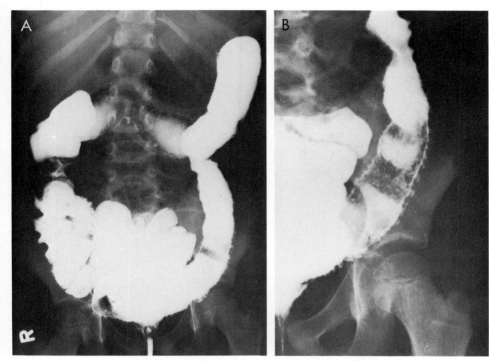

Fig 4–18.—Ulcerative colitis. **A,** frontal film from a barium enema reveals contrast material outside the lumen and in the wall, particularly evident in the descending colon. Note "collar-button" ulcerations. **B,** close-up shows the "collar-button" ulcerations to advantage. The key to diagnosis in this case is the abnormal *contour* of the bowel.

laterally to the left lower quadrant. The distal descending colon is seen at this level, with the proximal portions in the left flank and the left upper quadrant. Because of its contiguity with the spleen, the highest curve is noted as the splenic flexure. The transverse colon hangs from the mesentery in the midabdomen, suspended at the hepatic and splenic flexures. It is, as mentioned earlier, an anterior structure. The hepatic flexure is in the right upper quadrant and more caudad (inferior) than the splenic flexure. It lies just below the liver. The ascending colon is in the right lateral gutter, and its most proximal portion is the cecum. You can recognize it by detecting either the appendix or the ileocecal valve or by the reflux into the terminal ileum. The cecum is normally in the right lower quadrant overlying the iliac crest; when it lies between the iliac crest and the hepatic flexure, it may be mobile due to a loose fixation of the mesentery. However, when the cecum is not in the right lower quadrant, suspect the congenital abnormality mentioned above, malrotation or malfixation of the midgut (by definition, the midgut extends from the duodenal-jejunal junction to the splenic flexure, with the foregut being all bowel proximal to this and the hindgut being distal) (Fig 4–17).

The *contours* of the bowel lumen should be smooth and devoid of irregularities. When irregularities are present, they may be due to either poor preparation (retained fecal material) or pathologic conditions such as ulcerations of inflammatory bowel disease (Fig 4–18; compare Fig 4–16). The colon is normally indented at intervals by haustra or sacculations, which are smooth indentations caused by the

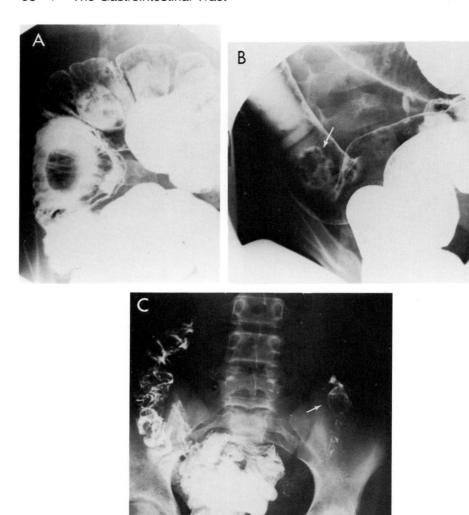

Fig 4–19.—Juvenile polyp of the colon. **A,** coned-down view of the ascending colon reveals a large lesion, well outlined by contrast medium. **B,** when the patient is positioned so that there is air in this portion of the colon, the lesion *(arrow)* is seen with its irregular margins. **C,** evacuation films are most helpful to show polypoid lesions. Note how a large juvenile polyp (on another patient) distends the otherwise collapsed descending colon *(arrow)*.

longitudinal muscular band on the surface of the colon that compresses it like an accordion. The muscles of the longitudinal band are called teniae coli. Normally, there are fewer haustral markings in the left colon than in the right.

After the colon has been filled and appropriate films taken, the patient is allowed to evacuate the contrast, and several postevacuation films (see Fig 4–16) are obtained to evaluate the mucosal pattern. On these films, the mucosa is feathery, and any mass within the colon, such as a polyp, disrupts this fine, regular, feathery pattern (Fig 4–19).

The *size* of the colon is greatest at the rectum and cecum. The left colon may be slightly smaller than the rest of the colon.

The search for intraluminal filling defects is mandatory at fluoroscopy and also on filled and postevacuation films. Since these may represent polyps, look for a stalk. The most common intraluminal filling defect in children is fecal material, but the most common pathologic intraluminal defect is that of a juvenile polyp (see Fig 4–19).

Since it is easier and faster to evacuate the contrast from the colon, the barium enema precedes the upper GI series when both are ordered for a gastrointestinal workup. A delay of several days may be involved if the upper GI is done before the enema. If ultrasound or radionuclide examination is indicated, these examinations should also precede the barium study.

EVALUATION OF OTHER ORGAN SYSTEMS WITHIN THE ABDOMEN

THE LIVER AND BILIARY SYSTEM

You have already noted liver size on the plain film and have indirectly determined if there was a mass arising from the liver by displacement of the stomach and duodenum. You have looked for calcifications within the liver and gallbladder. A more specific evaluation of the liver and biliary system would involve any of four new noninvasive imaging modalities: ultrasonography, radionuclide imaging, computerized tomography (CT scan), or nuclear magnetic resonance (NMR). The least invasive procedure is ultrasonography; therefore, we will discuss it fully. The ultrasound, CT, and NMR examinations provide precise anatomical information, while the radionuclide study gives only *gross* anatomical information but *precise* functional information.

Ultrasonic evaluation usually visualizes the liver in transverse and longitudinal sections. Transverse ultrasonic sections of the abdomen (as well as CT transverse sections) are oriented with the patient's right on the viewer's left; the superior aspect of the scan is the abdominal surface with the patient supine (Figs 4–20 and 4–21). In the longitudinal sections, the patient's head is oriented to the viewer's left (see Fig 4–20).

Each organ has its own reproducible parenchymal architecture. The lack of echoes or anechoic regions suggests a fluid-filled structure, such as a blood vessel or gallbladder. It is not the purpose of this text to review the interpretation of ultrasonic scans, but rather to portray the anatomy of the hepatobiliary system (see Fig 4–20). It is fair to say, however, that ultrasonic evaluation of the gallbladder is the best method for demonstrating gallstones.

The CT scan has the same orientation as the transverse sonographic study. More precise anatomical information is obtained, but at some "cost." The young patient

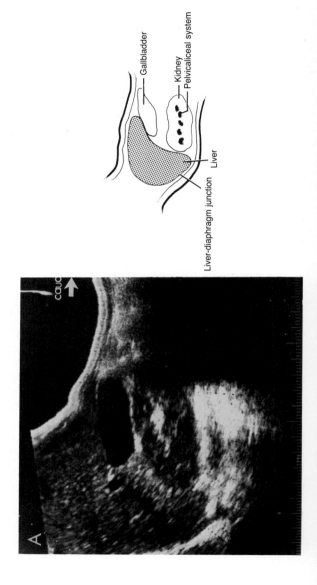

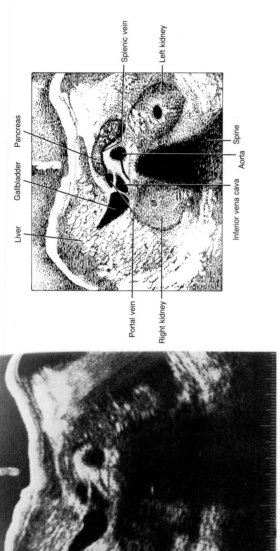

Fig 4–20.—Normal ultrasound. **A,** longitudinal section in the right upper quadrant (with schematic drawing) shows the liver-diaphragm interface, liver, gallbladder, and right kidney. **B,** transverse section of the upper abdomen shows the liver, gall-bladder, and pancreas anterior to the great vessels. The splenic vein runs behind the pancreas to reach the portal vein. The aorta is seen above the spine giving off the right renal artery, which passes behind the inferior vena cava to the right kidney.

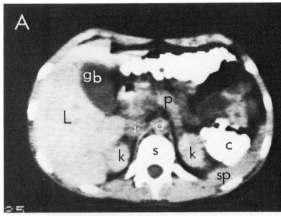

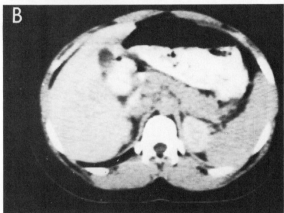

Fig 4–21.—CT scan of the upper abdomen. **A,** lower scan. *gb,* gallbladder; *L,* liver; *p,* pancreas; *c,* colon; *sp,* spleen; *s,* spine; *k,* kidney; *a,* aorta; *i,* inferior vena cava. **B,** upper scan. The barium in the gastrointestinal tract allows bowel to be differentiated from soft tissue masses. (Courtesy of Alkis Zingas, M.D.)

must be sedated, contrast medium must be injected for enhancement, bowel contrast must be utilized to opacify bowel loops for abdominal scans, and the study a priori uses X-radiation (see Fig 4–21).

An isotope scan of the liver is usually done with technetium bound to compounds taken up by either the reticuloendothelial system (technetium sulfur colloid) or hepatocytes (technetium iminodiacetic compounds). Sequential scans are obtained so that function can be properly assessed (Fig 4–22).

THE PANCREAS

Ultrasound is an excellent way of visualizing the pancreas. It is identified by finding some important anatomical landmarks (see Fig 4–20). The CT scan also demonstrates this area quite well (see Fig 4–21). There are no comparable radionuclide studies.

THE SPLEEN

The spleen can be seen by any of these three imaging modalities. However, nuclear medicine and CT scanning are preferred, particularly in cases of trauma, when both a functional and an anatomical evaluation are necessary.

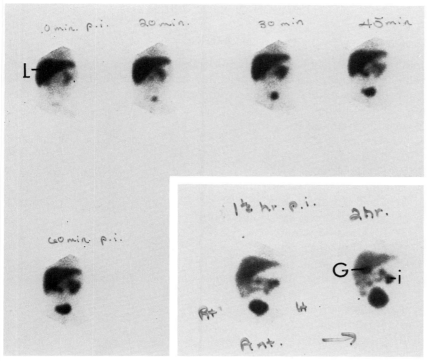

Fig 4–22.—Liver scan with technetium iminodiacetic compound, PIPIDA. Sequential scans show the isotope being taken up by the hepatocytes of the liver *(L)*, excreted into the gallbladder *(G)*, and eventually into the GI tract *(i)*. The liver intensity gradually diminishes. (Courtesy of Lawrence R. Kuhns, M.D.)

COMMON CLINICAL PROBLEMS

VOMITING

Vomiting is extremely common during childhood and is so nonspecific that history and physical examination are crucial to diagnosis. The character of the vomitus, as well as the age of the child, play an important role in the differential diagnosis, which is outlined below.

  I. Neonate to 2 months
      A. Nonbilious
          1. Chalasia
          2. Pyloric stenosis
      B. Bilious
          1. Small-bowel obstruction
              a. Small-bowel atresia (newborn)
              b. Midgut volvulus
          2. Hirschsprung's disease
 II. 2 months to 2 years
      A. Nonbilious (rarely an organic cause other than chalasia)
      B. Bilious
          1. Midgut volvulus
          2. Small-bowel obstruction
          3. Intussusception
III. Over 2 years
      Most causes not related to GI tract abnormalities

From age 1 day to 2 months, the most common cause of nonbilious vomiting is chalasia—gastroesophageal reflux. Immaturity of the esophagogastric junction results in food substances (or contrast during an esophagram) flowing back from the stomach into the esophagus. This obviously is diagnosed best during the fluoroscopic phase of the examination. The diagnosis can be made on the delayed film if there is contrast in the esophagus long after the patient has been given the barium. In most children, this is not accompanied by a hiatal hernia and is a self-limiting disorder.

Another common cause of nonbilious vomiting in this age group is pyloric stenosis (Fig 4–23). These children usually have projectile, nonbilious vomiting. If it persists for some time, the child will stop gaining weight, and electrolyte abnormalities (alkalosis with low chloride) will become apparent. On careful physical examination, the hypertrophied pyloric muscle can be palpated and feels somewhat like an olive. Most pediatric surgeons feel confident enough with this finding to operate and to reserve the gastrointestinal examination for the 10%–20% of patients in whom the finding is absent. The upper GI series defines the elongated, upturned curved pyloric canal with the "railroad track" and "teat" signs (see Fig 4–23).

In the neonate and infant up to 2 months of age, bilious vomiting strongly suggests obstruction distal to the entrance of the common bile duct into the duodenum. In the first day of life, atresias of the small bowel are suspected; and, using air as a contrast medium, the level of obstruction can be diagnosed by the number of air-filled, distended loops of bowel seen on the plain film (see Fig 4–11). Midgut volvulus is another important condition to consider. In these situations, there is

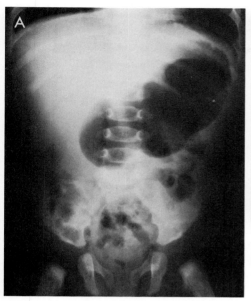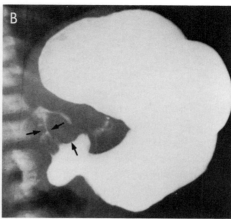

Fig 4–23.—Pyloric stenosis. **A,** supine film of the abdomen reveals distention of the stomach. Multiple peristaltic waves (contractions) are visible. This is one of the plain-film findings of gastric outlet obstruction. **B,** oblique view of this patient shows the elongated upturned pyloric channel with a single track (contrast in a compressed lumen) above the arrows, and a double, or railroad-track, configuration (contrast in two asymmetric lumens) below the arrows. In addition, there is an impression of the pyloric muscle on the base of the duodenal bulb and on the antral surface of the stomach *(single arrow).*

developmental abnormality of rotation and fixation of the midbowel from the ligament of Treitz to the splenic flexure. The ligament of Treitz is absent. Lack of proper fixation provides the mechanical basis that permits the bowel to twist (volvulus), leading to vascular compromise. Initially, venous return is occluded, followed by arterial obstruction involving the superior mesenteric artery (see Fig 4–16).

Causes of more distal abdominal obstruction presenting in the newborn include colonic atresia and aganglionosis (Hirschsprung's disease). In the latter, there is extensive dilatation of bowel loops, indicating low obstruction. When a barium enema is performed, a discrepancy between the *dilated proximal ganglionic portion* of bowel and the abnormal aganglionic distal portion of bowel is seen. The transition zone, together with the child's failure to satisfactorily evacuate the barium after 24 hours confirms the presence of mechanical bowel obstruction proximal to the malfunctioning colon segment.

Between 2 months and 2 years of age, the major cause of *nonbilious vomiting* continues to be chalasia (gastroesophageal reflux). *Bilious vomiting* in this age group suggests malrotation, small-bowel obstruction or intussusception. Intussusception occurs when small bowel invaginates into small bowel or colon, causing obstruction and eventual ischemia of the telescoped portion of the bowel—the intussusceptum (Fig 4–24). Most often, intussusception is manifest clinically by acute, colicky abdominal pain (see below) and in late stages by bloody diarrhea and signs of intes-

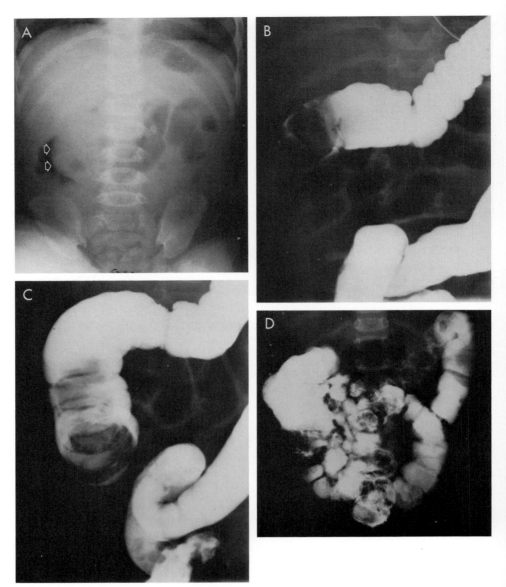

Fig 4–24.—Intussusception. **A,** Upright abdominal film in this 6-month-old with acute, colicky abdominal pain reveals a mass in the region of the hepatic flexure *(arrow)*. This finding was consistent on all films. **B,** a barium enema was done, and a large filling defect is seen in this region. **C,** this mass was then reduced by barium enema. **D,** there was abundant small-bowel reflux.

tinal obstruction. The obstruction often results in bilious vomiting.

In children over 2 years of age, most causes of vomiting are not related to GI tract anomalies, although certainly small-bowel obstruction, midgut volvulus, and intussusception do occur.

ABDOMINAL PAIN

This is an extremely common complaint in the pediatric age group. It can be separated into acute and chronic abdominal pain. In chronic abdominal pain, most clinicians have found radiographic studies (upper GI series and barium enema) are futile when pain is the only complaint. However, when this symptom is coupled with weight loss, diarrhea, and blood in the stool, inflammatory bowel disease is frequently found. The term "inflammatory bowel disease" includes regional enteritis and ulcerative colitis and can be diagnosed by various investigations of the upper and lower gastrointestinal tract (see Fig 4–17).

Acute abdominal pain in children is most often due to medical conditions such as gastroenteritis. However, the radiologist must be alert for surgical causes of abdominal pain, the most common of which are appendicitis, incarcerated inguinal hernia, and intussusception (see Figs 4–3, 4–10, 4–24). While routine plain radiography may be indicated when any of these conditions is suspected, only with an intussusception is the barium enema done. The radiographic signs of these three disorders are listed in Table 4–1.

BLUNT ABDOMINAL TRAUMA

Plain films of the abdomen may be extremely valuable in blunt abdominal trauma because free air, free fluid, sentinel loops, as well as fractured ribs and transverse processes of the spine can be found. Remember the radiologist's circle and ABCs. Injuries to the viscera are best defined by ultrasound and more invasive techniques, i.e., radionuclide imaging, CT scanning, angiography, etc.

CONSTIPATION

Late onset of symptoms, particularly after toilet training has begun, suggests a functional basis for this disorder. Plain-film studies reveal a dilated rectum and colon distended with stool. The barium enema confirms the presence of a large, capacious rectum, and postevacuation studies show *no lower segment* of narrowing.

However, if the patient has had a history of such difficulty from birth, one must

TABLE 4–1.—COMMON CAUSES OF ACUTE ABDOMINAL PAIN AND THEIR RADIOGRAPHIC SIGNS

DISEASE	RADIOGRAPHIC SIGNS
Appendicitis*	Appendicolith
	Free fluid in the cecal area or elsewhere within abdomen
	Sentinel loop of small bowel
	Absence of psoas margin
	Scoliosis, with concavity toward side of disorder
Inguinal hernia	Signs of intestinal obstruction
	Bowel gas in inguinal canal or lower
Intussusception†	Mass
	Signs of obstruction
	Coiled-spring appearance on barium enema

*In appendicitis, radiographic signs are found in only 50% of cases.
†A negative plain film should not deter one from doing a barium enema in a child with a clinical picture of intussusception.

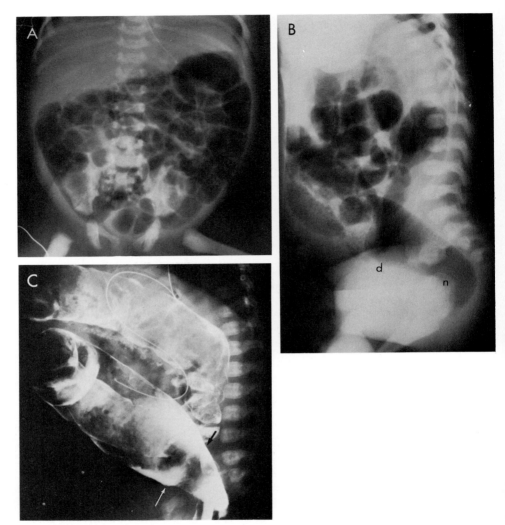

Fig 4–25.—Hirschsprung's disease. **A,** abdominal film in a 5-day-old reveals considerable distention of the bowel, with gas all the way down to the pelvis. **B,** on lateral films, the rectum is considerably smaller than any portion of the colon, and there is a transition zone between the nondilated
(n) and dilated *(d)* portions of the bowel. **C,** lateral postevacuation film reveals that the rectum is not
the most dilated portion of the colon. Arrows point to the transition zone between the nondistensible,
aganglionic distal colon and the dilated, ganglionic proximal colon. Note how much of the colon is
dilated. The rectum is unable to distend.

consider a diagnosis of Hirschsprung's disease (Fig 4–25). The barium enema will
demonstrate the findings of chronic mechanical obstruction from a malfunctioning
distal aganglionic segment. This may be most graphically seen on the postevacuation films, where the caliber disparity is striking. Since the examination is attempt-
ing to show not only anatomical abnormality but also pathophysiology, the usual
rigorous colonic emptying, i.e., purgatives and enemas, should be omitted.

RECTAL BLEEDING

Rectal bleeding varies from guaiac positive stools to frank bright-red blood. There are many causes, and the proper approach is determined by the suspected etiology in each case. Table 4–2 outlines the procedures

JAUNDICE

In the newborn, *prolonged* jaundice is most commonly due to either neonatal hepatitis or biliary atresia. None of the imaging procedures satisfactorily separates these two entities. However, ultrasonic examination is the initial procedure of choice, as it reveals any masses in the porta hepatis, such as a choledochal cyst. The second imaging procedure of choice is a radionuclide investigation (HIDA or PIPIDA) for the patency of the biliary system. At this writing, it seems that most children with prolonged jaundice undergo percutaneous liver biopsy. If the results of this biopsy show signs of obstructive liver disease, an exploratory laparotomy follows.

In older children with jaundice, the most common diagnosis is viral hepatitis. These children do not need roentgenographic evaluation, except when their course is atypical or recurrent. In these instances, ultrasound is an excellent, noninvasive method. Both gallstones and masses in the porta hepatis can be diagnosed. Intrahepatic biliary ductal obstruction with enlarged biliary radicals is easily seen. In the atypical case, procedures such as radionuclide study, CT scanning, percutaneous transhepatic cholangiography, and endoscopic retrograde duct catheterization may be necessary.

Figures 4–26 through 4–29 are presented as "unknowns." The history is given with each figure, and you are to make the correct diagnosis.

TABLE 4–2.—RECTAL BLEEDING

SUSPECTED CAUSES	KIND OF BLEEDING	PROCEDURE OF CHOICE
Peptic ulcer	Melena	Endoscopy and/or upper GI
Anal fissure	Blood-streaked stool	None; physical examination
Polyps	Red blood mixed with stool	Endoscopy and barium enema
Intussusception	See abdominal pain and vomiting in text	Barium enema with attempted hydrostatic reduction
Meckel's diverticulum	Voluminous, bright-red blood	Technetium radionuclide study
Inflammatory bowel disease	Bright red blood and/or streaking in stool	Endoscopy, upper GI with small-bowel follow-through, barium enema
Necrotizing enterocolitis (in newborns)	Variable	Plain films. Radiographic signs are: dilated bowel loops pneumatosis intestinalis (air out of bowel lumen but in wall of the bowel) portal venous gas free air

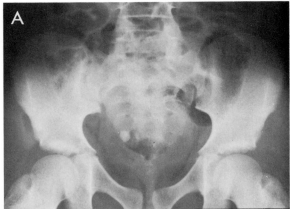

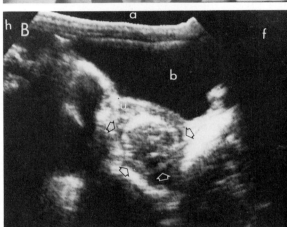

Fig 4–26.—Nine-year-old with abdominal pain. (See Appendix 2.)

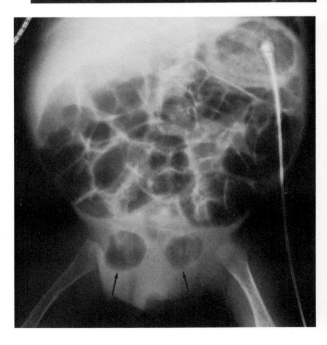

Fig 4–27.—An infant with abdominal distention. (See Appendix 2.)

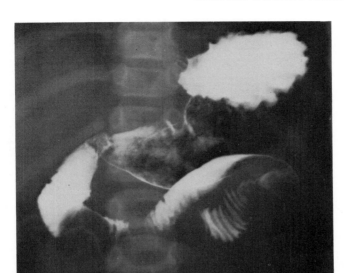

Fig 4–28.—Abdominal pain after trauma. (See Appendix 2.)

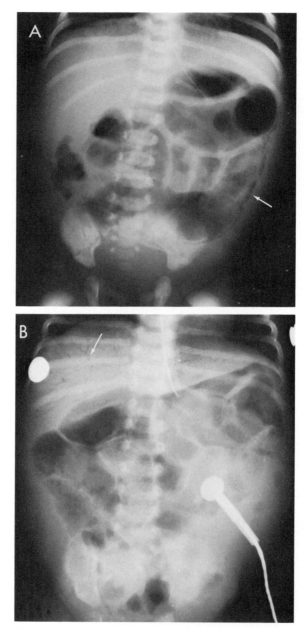

Fig 4–29.—Two neonates with abdominal distention. (See Appendix 2.)

SUGGESTED READING

1. Franken E.A., Jr.: *Gastrointestinal Radiology in Pediatrics*, ed. 2. Hagerstown, Md., Harper & Row, 1982.
2. Singleton E.G., Wagner M.L., Dulton R.V.: *Pediatric Radiology of the Alimentary Canal in Infants and Children.* Philadelphia, W. B. Saunders Co., 1977.

CHAPTER 5

The Urinary Tract

ROENTGENOGRAPHIC EVALUATION of the urinary tract in children begins with an abdominal radiograph. The lower urinary tract is studied next by means of a voiding cystourethrogram (VCU), followed by an intravenous injection of contrast material—the intravenous urogram (IVU). The newer modalities of ultrasound, radionuclide imaging, and computerized tomography, however, are rapidly earning a prominent, and in some cases primary, role in urinary tract imaging of children. Integration of these modalities will be discussed at the end of the chapter.

THE PLAIN FILM

Evaluation of the urinary tract begins with a plain film (see Chap. 4), which must show the diaphragm as well as the pubic bones. If this film does not include the entire abdomen, valuable information may be lost (Fig 5–1). You should use the systematic approach described in previous chapters to evaluate this film. When you see calcification, it is imperative to decide if it is within the urinary system. Oblique radiographs can facilitate your decision, since, once contrast material is injected, calcific densities may be obscured and precise localization will be difficult (see Fig 5–1).

Renal size can often be estimated from the plain film. A rough guide to appropriate size is that the length from the top to the bottom of the kidney should be no greater than 4–4½ vertebral bodies. The left kidney is usually slightly larger than the right (no greater than 1.5 cm difference). A kidney longer than 5 vertebral bodies is enlarged. The lower limits of normal are not as precise, but a kidney less than three vertebral bodies in length is abnormally small.

THE VCU

The purposes of the VCU are (1) to study the bladder and urethra for abnormalities of *size, position,* and *contour;* (2) to screen for vesicoureteral reflux (retrograde flow of contrast material into the ureters and/or kidneys); (3) to evaluate pelvic abnormalities that impinge on the bladder.

If the VCU is to be done alone, no preparation is necessary. The patient is asked to void, and then a small catheter (either a feeding tube or straight catheter) is placed through the urethra into the bladder. Residual urine is drained and the amount recorded. This is important because bladder dysfunction or distal obstruction can lead to retention after voiding. Contrast material is then instilled through the catheter into the bladder until it is filled to capacity.

The bladder appears as a round, opaque density, symmetrically situated in the pelvis. The inferior margin of the filled bladder should be seen at the top of the pubic symphysis on a well-centered film. The bladder wall is smooth, and there

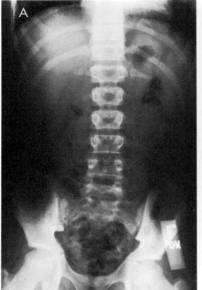 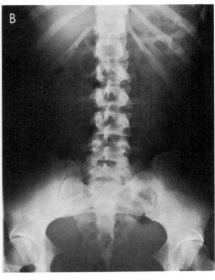

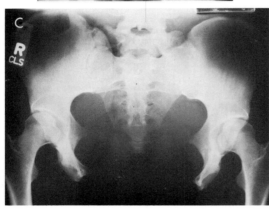

Fig 5–1.—Preliminary films. **A,** supine radiograph includes the bases of the lungs, the diaphragm, and the pubic bones. After the ABCs of the film are evaluated, try to note renal size. Did you note the hypoplasia of the right 12th rib? **B,** preliminary film of a 12-year-old girl. Is it adequate? **C,** pelvis of the young lady in **B** who has widespread pubic bones and had extrophy of the bladder. Did you see these findings in **B?** B included neither the diaphragm nor the pubic bones.

should be no filling defects within the bladder. Irregularity of the wall may indicate mucosal edema or diverticulum formation. Contrast seen in the ureters signifies incompetence of the ureterovesicle junction and reflux (Fig 5–2). When the catheter is removed, the patient voids, allowing for visualization of the urethra. This is much more crucial in a male, as significant pathology may exist in the posterior urethra, which is between the bladder neck and the urogenital diaphragm (see Fig 5–2). It is arbitrarily divided into the prostatic urethra and membranous urethra. In the male, the prostatic and ejaculatory ducts terminate in the verumontanum, located on the posterior wall of the prostatic urethra. The membranous urethra is shorter, beginning at the inferior margin of the veru and extending downward to the urogenital diaphragm. The anterior urethra extends from the urogenital diaphragm distally to the urethral meatus and is divided into the bulbous and penile portions. When there are abnormalities such as posterior urethral valves, there is marked discrepancy between the anterior and posterior urethral caliber (Fig 5–3).

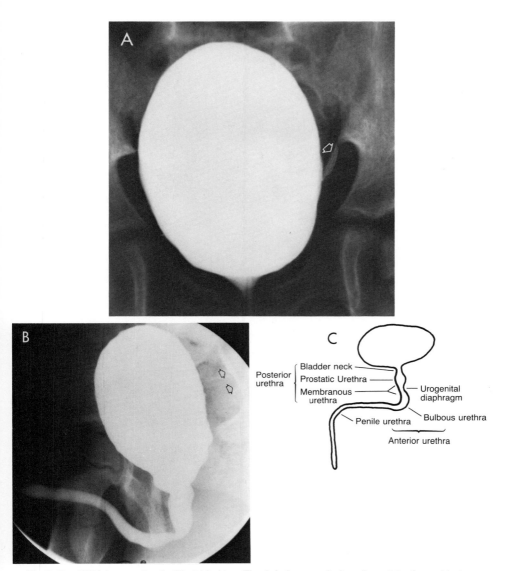

Fig 5–2.—VCU in a male. **A,** filled bladder. The inferior margin is adjacent to the pubic bones, and the bladder is in the center of the pelvis. There is no mass impression on the bladder. Contour and position are smooth and normal. Incidentally noted is a small amount of contrast in the distal left ureter (arrow). **B,** patient is placed in the oblique position, and the reflux into the left ureter is noted (arrows). After patient voids, the entire posterior urethra is easily seen; and, in this instance, the anterior urethra is seen as well. Slight irregularity at the base of the bladder posteriorly is expected during voiding. **C,** drawing of the male urethra.

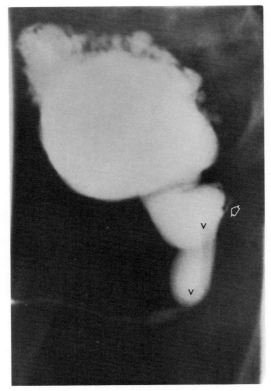

Fig 5–3.—Posterior urethral valves. This single oblique view during a VCU reveals the irregularity of the bladder wall. Large collections of contrast in saccules are due to bladder obstruction. The posterior urethra is quite dilated when compared to the anterior urethra. A line *(v)* representing the valve can be seen from the verumontanum to the region of the urogenital diaphragm. Note that the opening between the anterior and posterior urethra is located quite posteriorly and, of course, is narrowed (see normal urethra in Fig 5–2). Reflux into the ejaculatory ducts is also present *(arrow)*.

In the female, the urethra is shorter and is infrequently the site of significant pathology (Fig 5–4). Voiding in the recumbent position often causes vaginal filling, which is not pathologic.

During fluoroscopy, the upper abdomen is viewed to make sure there is no evidence of reflux of contrast material from the bladder to the kidneys (see Fig 5–2). This is important because reflux (of either infected or sterile urine) can cause parenchymal atrophy, frequently most marked in the polar regions. A postvoiding film is obtained to see if the bladder empties completely.

In instances of trauma to the pelvis, the possibility of urethral disruption must be considered. This anterior portion of the urethra is best seen when a small catheter is placed within the urethral meatus and retrograde injection is made. If the urethra is intact, the catheter is passed into the bladder and a conventional VCU is done to visualize the posterior urethra.

What abnormalities do you see in Figure 5–5? (Answer in Appendix.)

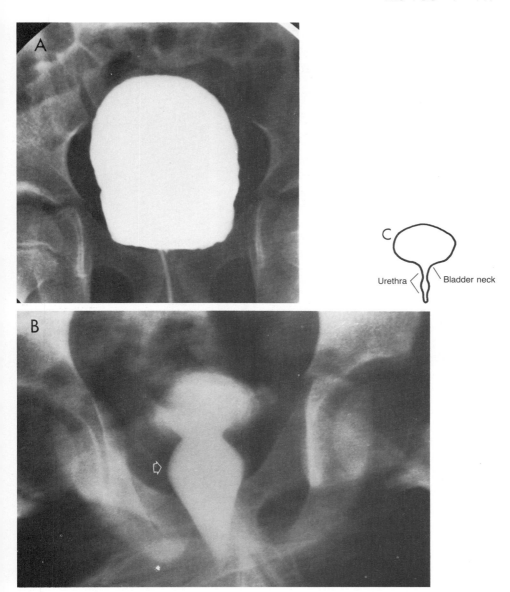

Fig 5–4.—The female urethra. **A,** filled bladder with catheter in place again reveals the central position of the bladder without any mass impinging on its wall. **B,** on voiding, the posterior aspect of the bladder becomes slightly irregular. The urethra is much shorter in a female and often displays a "carrot-top" or "spinning-top" deformity *(arrow).* There is often reflux into the vagina when the patient voids in the recumbent position. **C,** drawing of the female urethra.

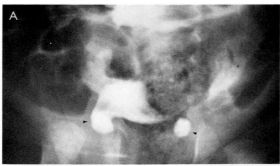

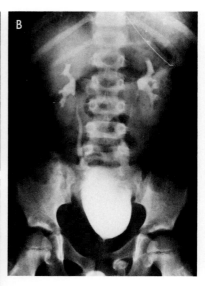

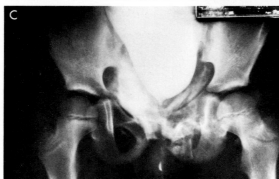

Fig 5–5.—What abnormalities do you see? (Answers in Appendix 2.)

THE IVU

INDICATIONS

Patients with any of the following conditions should have an IVU included in their work-up:

Urinary tract infection

Abdominal mass (see Chap. 6)

Hematuria of unknown etiology

Renal or bladder trauma

Recurrent abdominal pain with clinical evidence of urinary tract disease

Conditions that predispose to renal tumors (tuberous sclerosis, hemihypertrophy, Beckwith's syndrome, aniridia)

Failure to thrive

Meningomyelocele

Malformations associated with a moderate to high degree of renal anomalies (unusual development of the ears, imperforate anus, anomalies of the reproductive system, unexplained or refractory pneumomediastinum or pneumothorax in the newborn, fetal alcohol syndrome). (Ultrasound is also sufficient to rule out malformations.)

TECHNIQUE

As opposed to the passive instillation of contrast material in the VCU, tri-iodin-ated benzoic acid derivatives are injected intravenously as an active imaging agent in the IVU. This hyperosmolar (1,200–1,500 mosm/L) agent is filtered by the glomeruli and collects in the renal tubules, affording an insensitive evaluation of renal function; little change in degree of opacification is seen until there is major elevation of the serum creatinine level.

Problems with intravenous injection of iodinated contrast medium include allergic reactions, renal shutdown secondary to the precipitation of Tamm-Horsfall protein in the kidneys (especially if the patient is dehydrated), and congestive heart failure because of the hyperosmolar effect of the contrast material. Obviously, then, special precautions must be taken before the IVU with children who are dehydrated, who have a history of allergic reaction to iodides, or who have leukemia or lymphoma and are prone to have elevated uric acid levels.

Proper preparation of the patient is important so that the kidneys can be optimally visualized and the effects of the contrast material minimized. Premedication of allergic patients is of questionable value, but avoiding significant dehydration before injecting contrast material is crucial. In addition, cleansing the colon improves visualization of the kidneys, so a cathartic or single enema is frequently given.

In general (after a preliminary film), the IVU consists of an early or *nephrogram* film exposed at 30–60 seconds after injection, with subsequent frontal films taken 5 to 15 minutes after injection. (One of these may be a postvoiding film.) Oblique and/or lateral films are added as needed. Each film has a specific role in evaluation of the urinary tract.

THE NEPHROGRAM

This film (Fig 5–6) is taken about 1 minute after injection of contrast medium (after the neonatal period, 1 cc/lb up to 50 lbs). As the contrast circulates through the arteries and capillaries, the vascular portions of the body become opacified (total body opacification—TBO effect); and avascular areas such as cysts and hydronephrotic kidneys are highlighted (Fig 5–7). The film is taken with the patient prone and is coned down to the kidneys and upper abdomen (unless we are studying another area of the body). This is the best film on which to see the renal parenchyma.

Here we are studying *size, contour,* and *position* of the kidneys. The normal *size* of the kidneys (Table 5–1) has already been mentioned—between 4 and 5 vertebral bodies.

The *contour* of the kidneys should be smooth or smoothly indented incident to fetal lobulation, in sharp contrast to the abrupt scarring noted at sites of pyelonephritis or reflux atrophy. The parenchyma normally should be equal in all areas of the kidney.

The *position* of the kidney should be obliquely oriented so that the upper pole is closer to the spine than the lower pole, and the kidney should lie just lateral to the psoas muscle margin. Any deviation is indicative of a mass until proved otherwise. The kidney, at this point, should appear homogeneous, with no difference between the density of the inner surface and the outer surface. On direct lateral projection, the kidneys overlie the spine.

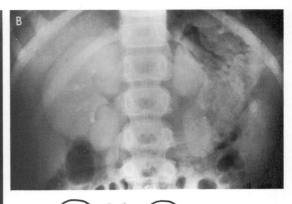

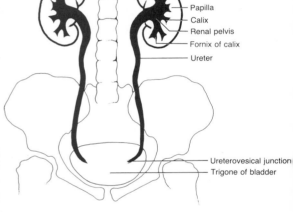

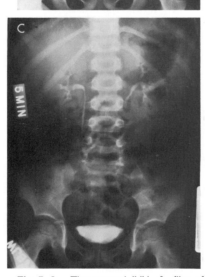

Renal cortex
Papilla
Calix
Renal pelvis
Fornix of calix
Ureter

Ureterovesical junction
Trigone of bladder

Fig 5–6.—The normal IVU. **A,** film of the abdomen, including both the diaphragms and pubic bones. Use the systematic approach to evaluate this film! **B,** prone, coned-down view shows a nephrogram effect. The kidneys are homogeneous at this point, and there is very little contrast material in the collecting systems. Occasionally, such a film is taken several minutes after injection; and then the collecting systems will be seen to better advantage. On this initial film, the renal axis is noted with the upper pole being closer to the spine than the lower pole. The renal contours are evaluated and should be smooth without scarring or indentations. **C,** 5-minute film reveals the renal collecting systems, the calices, and the infundibulum leading to the renal pelvis. Any deviation or blunting of the collecting system is seen at this time. The renal pelvis then tapers into the ureter. The ureters pass inferiorly, crossing the margins of the transverse processes. The bladder is separate from the pubic bones because it is partially filled. A 10-minute frontal film is usually obtained to view the entire system to see if there has been any change secondary to osmotic load. **D,** drawing of the normal intrarenal anatomy as seen on the IVU.

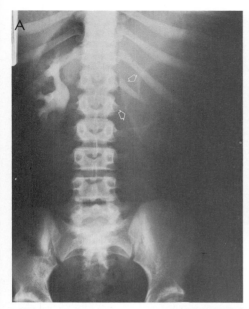

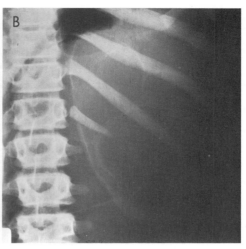

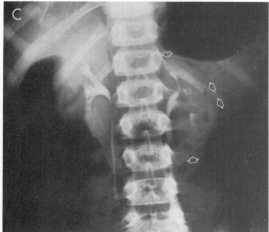

Fig 5–7.—Multiple abnormal IVUs. (See Appendix 2.)

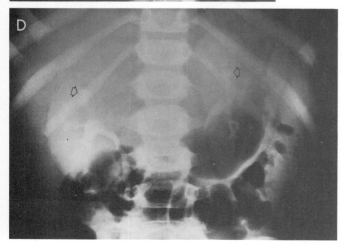

121

TABLE 5–1.—DIFFERENTIAL DIAGNOSIS
RELATIVE TO SIZE OF KIDNEY ON IVU

I. Large Kidneys
  A. Single large kidney
    Tumor
    Renal vein thrombosis
    Pyelonephritis
    Abscess
    Hematoma
    Obstruction
  B. Two large kidneys
    Polycystic disease
    Hydronephrosis due to neurogenic
    bladder, posterior urethral valves, or
    other obstruction
    Glycogen storage disease
    Amyloid
    Bilateral Wilms' tumor
    Acute glomerulonephritis
II. Small Kidneys
  A. Single small kidney
    Chronic renal disease
    Congenital hypoplastic kidney (renal
    artery stenosis)
    Reflux
  B. Two small kidneys
    Chronic renal insufficiency
    Reflux
III. Non-visualized Kidney
    Congenital absence of the kidney
    Surgically removed kidney
    Ectopic kidney
    Renal artery thrombosis
    Renal vein thrombosis
    Tumor

THE 5–15-MINUTE FILMS

By this time, the contrast material has filtered from the vascular system, through the glomeruli, and into the renal collecting systems. A streaking of contrast material in the renal tubules leading into the renal papilla may be seen; it is called the tubular blush. The delicate fornices of the calix and the infundibula are seen leading to the renal pelves (see Fig 5–6). If you draw an outline of the lateral aspect of the kidney and then a line connecting the tips of the fornices of each calix, the two semicircles should be concentric. If they are not, suspect loss of parenchyma, with the calix extending closer to the outer margin of the kidney. In this way also, you can see how much parenchyma is medial to the most medial calix of the superior pole. This polar region is a common site of parenchymal loss in reflux nephropathy. Similarly, the distance from the lower calices to the spine should be checked for parenchymal loss. There may be a vascular impression on either the fornix, calix, or renal pelvis. On multiple views, these can be identified as vascular changes by their tubular contour.

Next, inspect the renal pelvis and ureters. The renal pelvis may be intrarenal or extrarenal (inside or outside the renal contour). If the pelvis is extrarenal, it tends to be larger and more easily distensible with osmotic loads. However, even in those instances, the calices remain normal. The renal pelvis tapers at the ureteropelvic junction into the proximal ureter. As the ureters descend to the pelvis, they generally overlie the transverse processes of the spine. If they do not, a medial mass (enlarged lymph nodes, etc.) should be suspected. Oblique and lateral views are helpful in this situation. Once again, we are looking at *size, contour,* and *position* when we view the ureters. Frequently as the bladder fills, the upper tracts become dilated.

DELAYED FILMS

REED'S RULE #11—During intravenous urography, keep taking films as long as you are getting needed information.

When there are abnormalities of the urinary system, delayed visualization of the kidney's collecting system is not uncommon. In instances of urinary tract obstruction, hypotension, or abnormal handling of the contrast, 12-, 24-, and 48-hour films are helpful. Normally, 50% of the contrast is excreted in 2 hours, and all is gone within 24 hours. When taking delayed films, supine, prone, and lateral views may be selectively requested until the entire system is visualized. The value of the prone film is that the more anterior structures—renal pelvis and ureter—may be aided by gravity and fill to better advantage.

When a kidney is obstructed, the collecting system distends at the expense of the parenchyma. The more chronic the obstruction, the greater the distention. The parenchyma is compressed, with the tubules assuming a more nearly horizontal orientation. Thus, during the early phase, the urine-filled calices are lucent, and the tubules form a parenchymal rim (see Fig 5–7). As the delayed films are obtained, the collecting system slowly fills. Contrast accumulates along the outer portion of the fluid-filled calix, forming a calyceal crescent. Prone films are very helpful.

What abnormalities can you detect on the different IVUs in Figure 5–7?

Evaluation of the neonatal urinary system is somewhat more difficult. In the first week or two of life, the neonate's renal blood flow, glomerular filtration rate, and renal tubule concentrating ability are decreased, compared to that of older infants. For these reasons, other imaging modalities, such as ultrasound or radionuclide imaging, are frequently utilized. Nonetheless, it is possible to get an adequate IVU of the neonate if the following modifications are made. The study must be prolonged; that is, the ability to see the kidneys in the nephrogram phase and collecting systems must be delayed so that a good nephrogram may be seen at 5–10 minutes. Films over 30–90 minutes may be necessary for optimal visualization of the renal pelvis and ureters. In addition, it may be crucial to order tomograms and/or a lateral film because renal outlines may be obscured by gas on the frontal projection (Fig 5–8).

The neonate is a prime example of the need to specifically tailor the urogram. Another example is the neurologically impaired child with abundant fecal material in the colon; he is uncooperative and may need a specific form of bowel preparation. Under some of these circumstances, oblique projections, tomographic studies, or delayed films are mandatory.

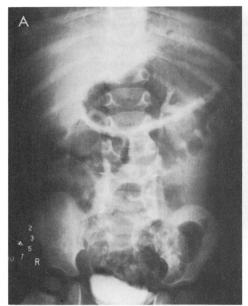

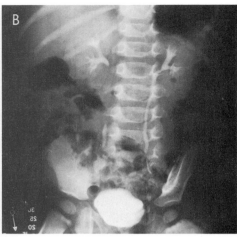

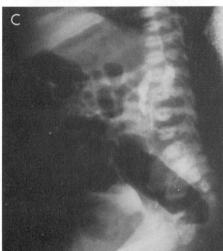

Fig 5–8.—Normal neonatal IVU. **A,** supine film of an IVU in a neonate with ambiguous genitalia. It is difficult to see both kidneys well. **B, C,** additional films, prone and lateral, help to visualize the collecting systems.

ULTRASOUND

Ultrasound is a method by which high-frequency (3.5–10 megahertz) sound waves are used to evaluate internal anatomical structures. It is an *anatomical*, not a physiologic, evaluation. As the sound beam encounters different normal renal structures (cortex, medulla, etc.) differences in acoustics are reflected back to a transducer and displayed on a television monitor (Fig 5–9). There are two types of ultrasound—static and real-time examination. Static examination is similar to plain-film radiography in that a single static picture of the organ is obtained for evaluation. Real-time sonography is similar to fluoroscopy in that it records the motion of

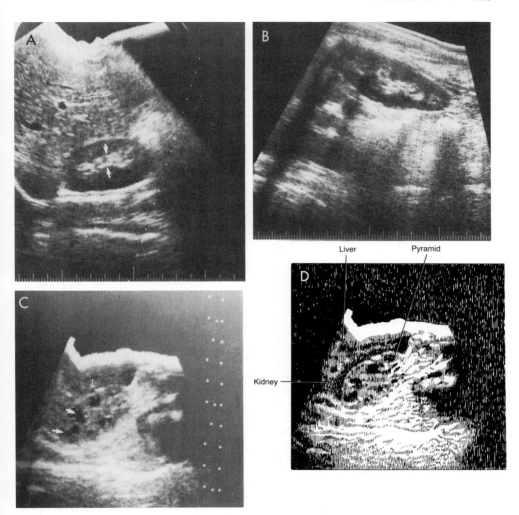

Fig 5–9.—Ultrasonic evaluation of the kidneys. **A,** supine longitudinal ultrasound scan shows that the renal parenchyma in an older child is less echogenic than the liver, and there are bright central sinus echoes *(arrows)* in the renal collecting systems because of peripelvic fat. **B,** prone scan in an older child shows the central collecting system and a few of the medullary rays, which are not as obvious in older children as they are in the neonate. **C,** neonatal longitudinal scan of the right kidney shows no central sinus echoes. There is increased echogenicity of the renal cortex in relation to the liver *(L),* with prominent pyramids *(arrows).* **D,** drawing of ultrasonic anatomy.

various organs. Ureteral peristalsis and dynamic bladder emptying may be imaged as these events occur. It is particularly useful in cases of urinary tract obstruction. For example, if the kidney is hydronephrotic, the obstruction may lie at the junction of the kidney and ureter, at the junction of the ureter and bladder, or even more distally. Real-time sonography allows you to scan the abdomen for the point at which the ureters are no longer dilated and, therefore, to determine the point of obstruction without delayed films or active contrast.

Since there is no injection of contrast material and the kidneys can almost always

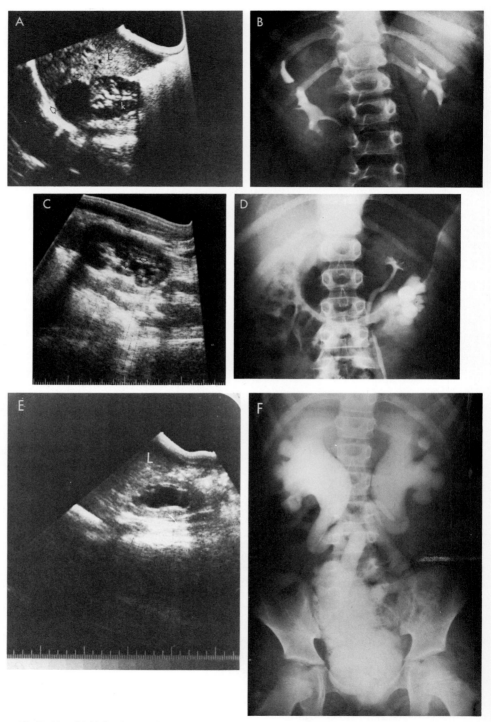

Fig 5–10.—Multiple abnormalities detected on ultrasound. What do you see? (Answers in Appendix 2.)

be viewed despite bowel gas, no patient preparation is needed for the ultrasound examination.

Multiple views of the kidneys are obtained in transverse, oblique, and longitudinal planes. The patient is studied in both supine, prone, and coronal positions, and normal renal architecture is readily discernible (see Fig 5–9). The fluid-filled portions of the kidney—the medullary rays and dilated central sinus collecting systems—appear anechoic, i.e., without echoes. The cortex has a distinctive architectural pattern with some internal echoes but distinctly fewer echoes than the liver (except in neonates). Echogenic peripelvic fat helps to delineate this region (the CSE—central sinus echoes).

What abnormalities do you see in Figure 5–10?

RADIONUCLIDE IMAGING

Radioactive substances such as technetium-99 pertechnetate may be bound to various compounds to give a radionuclide, which is injected intravenously. When the target organ takes up this compound in a normal physiological manner, the

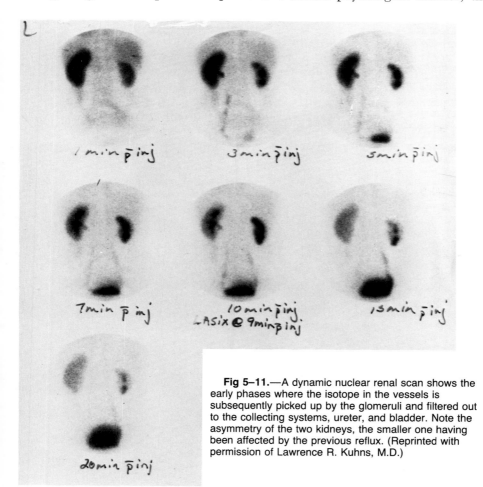

Fig 5–11.—A dynamic nuclear renal scan shows the early phases where the isotope in the vessels is subsequently picked up by the glomeruli and filtered out to the collecting systems, ureter, and bladder. Note the asymmetry of the two kidneys, the smaller one having been affected by the previous reflux. (Reprinted with permission of Lawrence R. Kuhns, M.D.)

radioactive emissions help to indicate the physiology and function of the organ of interest.

For example, ^{99m}Tc is labeled to such chelates as DTPA (diethylenetriamine penta-acetic acid) and DMSA (dimercaptosuccinic acid). The former is handled by glomerular filtration, and the latter by the tubules. Renal function can be precisely evaluated when the imaging technique is coupled to a sophisticated computer analysis. A dynamic scan shows the vascular uptake of the radionuclide as well as parenchymal handling of the radionuclide. Sedation may be required to insure patient immobility, since renal processing of the compound proceeds over a period of time. The radiation dose from these procedures is low.

These data are usually sufficient to evaluate unilateral renal function and to compare the two sides (Fig 5–11). The radionuclide study is the most precise evaluation of renal function we have in our imaging armamentarium. It can detect abnormalities of function well before the IVU.

COMPUTERIZED TOMOGRAPHY

This imaging modality provides precise anatomical evaluation. In addition, it allows one to view adjacent viscera within the abdomen that may involve the kidneys. Since the patient must be immobilized for varying amounts of time, most children under 5 years of age will have to be sedated. Intravenous contrast is given during the examination to help visualize the kidneys. The dose of contrast is greater than that used in intravenous urography. This procedure has the highest radiation dose of those discussed.

Figure 5–12 shows the exquisite detail obtained with CT scanning. In this ex-

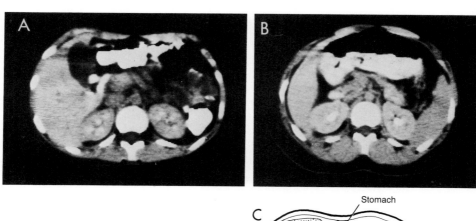

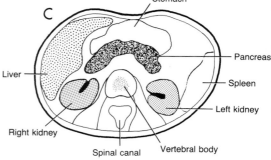

Fig 5–12.—A normal CT scan of the kidneys. **A,** upper scan. **B,** lower scan. **C,** drawing of CT. (Reprinted with permission of Alkis Zingas, M.D.)

ample, you are looking at cross-sectional anatomy as seen on abdominal ultrasound. With the newer machines, utilizing gathered mathematical data, longitudinal reconstruction of the image can be performed.

INTEGRATION OF THE IMAGING MODALITIES

The basic questions to ask before ordering an imaging modality of the urinary tract are:

1. Why am I doing this study?
2. What do I hope to learn?
3. Am I after an anatomical evaluation (i.e., tumor, anomaly, or obstruction) or a functional evaluation (i.e., decreased renal function)?

An appropriate imaging modality can only be selected after your goals are clear in your mind. Table 5–2 summarizes these modalities. The decision as to which imaging modality one selects is really a tradeoff. If you are screening or looking for a low-yield abnormality, the procedure with the least radiation and least danger that can give you the answer is appropriate. It is for this reason that ultrasound frequently is selected as the first imaging modality. On the other hand, if you are evaluating a tumor of the abdomen or the kidney, the most precise information is crucial; therefore, computed tomographic studies are frequently utilized. The four imaging modalities discussed in this chapter may be complementary. For example, an anechoic lesion on ultrasound may be a renal cyst, hydronephrosis, or a duplicated kidney. Only by correlating this finding with intravenous urography can the correct diagnosis be made (Fig 5–13).

Two other modalities should be mentioned. Selective percutaneous renal arteriography shows vascular anatomy most precisely. It is an invasive procedure and is discussed in Chapter 9. A newer modality—digital angiography—is now available. After an intravenous injection, the data are processed by computer and renal vasculature can be visualized. The efficacy of digital angiography and NMR in children needs to be determined.

TABLE 5–2.—IMAGING MODALITIES

	UROGRAPHY	ULTRASOUND	NUCLEAR MEDICINE	COMPUTERIZED TOMOGRAPHY
Anatomy	+ +	+ +	+	+ + +
Function	+	−	+ + +	+
Radiation	Low	None	Low	Highest of group
Injection of contrast/ radionuclide	Yes	No	Yes	Yes
Patient preparation	Yes	No	No	Yes
Sedation under age 5	No	No	Probably	Probably

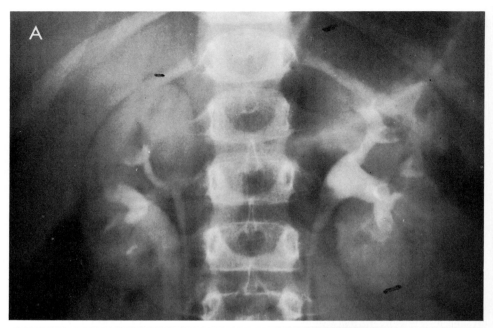

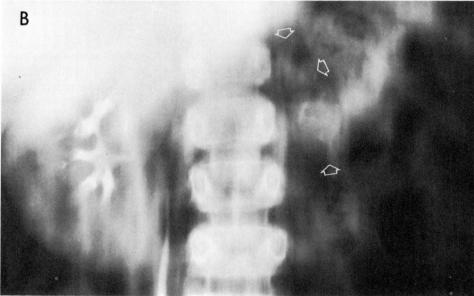

Fig 5–13.—A child with pyelonephritis and a child with reflux. **A,** this child was screened for a urinary tract infection. Note that the right kidney, which is smaller than the left, has a duplicated collecting system. The right lower pole parenchyma is thinner than the upper pole, and the ureter is dilated due to reflux that had been undetected for many years. (The kidneys are marked for size.) **B,** this child has a small shrunken left kidney that is best seen by this tomogram. The right kidney is compensatorily enlarged, but otherwise unremarkable.

COMMON CLINICAL SITUATIONS

INFECTION

Upper urinary tract infection must be documented before radiographic studies are requested. Although the presence of bacteria on Gram stains of a fresh, unspun, clean-catch specimen is very suggestive of a urinary tract infection, this must be confirmed with a quantitative urine culture. A colony count of 100,000 per milliliter of midstream voided specimen is considered a positive urine culture. The radiographic work-up proceeds after the patient has been treated. Imaging evaluation should be done because:

1. This is the *first diagnosed* urinary tract infection, not necessarily the *first actual* infection. Urinary tract infection may be missed for some time, and kidney damage may well be present.
2. You want to rule out underlying congenital anatomical abnormalities.

Both males and females are studied with a VCU followed by an IVU after the first documented urinary tract infection (see Fig 5–13). In some instances, an ultrasound examination, rather than an IVU, is done if the VCU is normal.

ENURESIS

Most nocturnal bedwetters do not require any imaging studies. Careful history taking, centering on the symptoms of urinary tract infection, neurogenic bladder, and persistent versus intermittent wetting, should clarify the problem. If the imaging work-up is pursued, a VCU and IVU (?ultrasound) are done to rule out anatomical changes of renal scarring, neurogenic bladder, and abnormalities such as an ectopic ureteral insertion.

ABDOMINAL MASS

This clinical phenomenon is discussed fully in Chapter 6.

HEMATURIA

Blunt abdominal trauma is a common cause of renal injury. When the trauma involves the upper abdomen, a urogram may be done as a gross evaluation of renal function and a precise evaluation of anatomical detail. Computerized tomographic studies give the best detail of the kidneys and adjacent visceral injury and, in some circumstances, may be the initial procedure. When there is injury to the lower abdomen and pelvis, a VCU, followed by an IVU, is obtained (remember, you may need to study the anterior urethra). At the same time, precise detail can be obtained with computerized tomography and contrast enhancement. The latter may be preferable because it avoids instrumentation of the urethra in an acutely injured patient.

In nontraumatic hematuria, the need for an imaging modality reflects the clinical diagnosis. Acute β-streptococcal glomerulonephritis or Henoch-Schönlein purpura are not indications for an IVU. However, since tumors can present with hematuria, a precise anatomical evaluation is appropriate if the diagnosis is uncertain. Because of the lower radiation dose and, in many instances, the ease of obtaining the examination, an IVU or an ultrasound scan is done first.

SUGGESTED READING

1. Swischuk L.E.: *Radiology of the Newborn and Young Infant,* ed. 2. Baltimore, Williams & Wilkins Co., 1980.
2. Caffey J.: *Pediatric X-ray Diagnosis,* ed. 7. Chicago, Year Book Medical Publishers, Inc., 1978.

CHAPTER 6

Abdominal and Pelvic Masses

THE PEDIATRICIAN frequently asks the pediatric radiologist to verify an abdominal or pelvic mass and to suggest possible diagnoses. The imaging approach to these problems varies, but these basic principles must be followed:

1. The initial procedure should be a three-view abdominal series (Chap. 4).
2. When there is only a *question* of a mass, the least invasive procedure should be done first.
3. Once a mass has been established, the work-up is guided by the patient's *age*, the *location of the mass*, and the *symptoms*.
4. The following priorities should be kept in mind:
   a. Since barium interferes with ultrasound, radionuclide imaging, CT, and IVUs, any barium examination should follow these three studies.
   b. If both a barium enema and an upper GI series are necessary, the barium enema should be done first because barium is more readily cleared from the colon.
5. The pediatric radiologist is the best source of information as to how the imaging work-up should proceed.

BEGIN THE WORK-UP WITH AN ABDOMINAL SERIES

Almost every child who presents with an abdominal mass should have abdominal films as an initial screening procedure (except for girls over 9 years of age, who may be pregnant). Plain-film findings and abdominal series have already been discussed in Chapters 4 and 5. Specifically, you should look for mass effects and calcifications.

Mass effect (see Fig 4–7) is the effect of the mass on contiguous structures, such as bowel or viscera. Divide the abdomen into quadrants and apply your knowledge of anatomical structures in this quadrant.

> REED'S RULE #12—Try to find the effects of the mass on adjacent organs on each abdominal film. Draw the mass, if necessary.

Calcifications (see Fig 4–5) are an important clue to the type of mass present. Fine, punctate calcifications next to the upper pole of the kidney may well represent an adrenal neuroblastoma, while coarse, large calcifications may merely mean the presence of calcified adrenal hemorrhage. It is common for the neuroblastoma to calcify, while it is distinctly less common for a Wilms' tumor to calcify. An appendicolith is ordinarily solitary and laminated, while a calcification in a dermoid or teratoma has a structure similar to teeth in the jaw. You must then decide where the mass originated and whether it is neoplastic, inflammatory, etc.

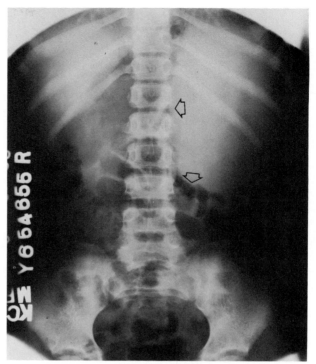

Fig 6–1.—Enlarged spleen. The gas-filled gastrointestinal tract is displaced inferiorly and to the right *(arrows)*. The differential diagnosis of anatomical origin for the mass includes muscle, peritoneum, kidney, spleen, adrenal gland, stomach and mesenteries. These are structures that are found "skin to skin." This child had isolated splenomegaly due to portal hypertension.

> *REED'S RULE #13—After you have defined the mass, find the center of the lesion. Then consider all structures, gross and microscopic, near the center of the lesion as possible sources of the mass. Think skin to skin.*

Remember, an abdominal mass may be an enlarged organ, such as the liver, spleen, or kidney. Frequently, children with leukemia have visceromegaly. Isolated splenomegaly is found in portal hypertension (Fig 6–1).

BEGIN WITH THE LEAST INVASIVE STUDY WHEN THERE IS A QUESTIONABLE MASS

Frequently, the clinician is not sure if there is a mass. In a constipated child, fecal masses in the colon are easily palpated and may be mistaken for a lesion. Other putative masses include the distended urinary bladder and the abdominal aorta in a particularly thin child. Therefore, evacuation of both bowel and bladder contents should precede any work-up to obviate the majority of "pseudomasses."

In the female over age 9, any pelvic mass should be considered an intrauterine pregnancy until proved otherwise. For this reason, ultrasound is initially utilized because it is the least invasive modality without ionizing radiation (Fig 6–2).

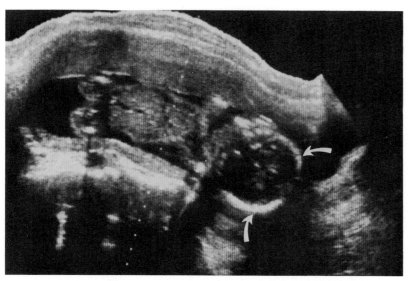

Fig 6–2.—Intrauterine pregnancy. This 11-year-old girl presented with a pelvic mass. Ultrasound revealed an intrauterine fetus. The arrows point to the fetal head.

TABLE 6–1.—Most Frequent Abdominal and Pelvic
Masses* by Age

AGE AND TYPE OF MASS	INCIDENCE (%)
Neonate	
Renal	55 ⎫
Hydronephrosis	⎬ 70%
Multicystic kidney	⎪
Genital	15 ⎭
Hydrometrocolpos	
Ovarian	
Gastrointestinal	15
Duplications	
Volvulus	
Nonrenal retroperitoneal	10
Adrenal hemorrhage	
Neuroblastoma	
Teratoma	
Hepatosplenobiliary	5
One Month to Two Years	
Renal	55 ⎫
Wilms' tumor	⎬ 78%
Hydronephrosis	⎪
Nonrenal retroperitoneal	23 ⎭
Neuroblastoma	
Teratoma	
Gastrointestinal (including biliary masses and	18
appendiceal abscess) and intussusception	
Genital, miscellaneous	4
Older Than Two Years†	
Visceromegaly secondary to infection, leukemia,	Frequent†
lymphoma, splenomegaly secondary to portal	Frequent†
hypertension	
Wilms' tumor and neuroblastoma	Frequent to age 5; decreases thereafter†
Appendiceal abscess	Frequent over age 2
Intussusception	Most frequent at age 2; decreases thereafter†
Pregnancy	Most common pelvic mass in females over age 9†

*Modified from: Griscom N.T.: The roentgenology of neonatal abdominal masses. *A.J.R.* 93:447, 1965; Kasper T.E., et al.: Urological abdominal masses in infants and children. *J. Urol.* 116:629, 1976; Melicow M.D. and Uson A.C.: Palpable abdominal masses in infants and children: A report based on review of 653 cases. *J. Urol.* 81:705, 1959.

†It is difficult to obtain precise numbers for this age group.

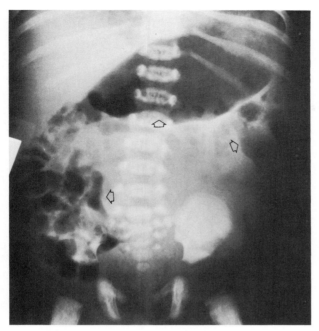

Fig 6–3.—Ovarian cyst. This 6-month-old girl presented with a central lower abdominal mass. The plain film of the abdomen reveals bowel displaced away from this mass *(arrows)*. Pelvic masses, when they enlarge, leave the true pelvis and are found in the infraumbilical region. At surgery, this proved to be a large ovarian cyst. The arrows indicate the "mass effects."

LET THE PATIENT'S AGE, SYMPTOMS, AND LOCATION OF THE MASS DIRECT THE WORK-UP (TABLE 6–1)

NEWBORN

Seventy percent of the abdominal and pelvic masses in neonates originate in the genitourinary tract. Hydronephrosis and multicystic kidneys account for the majority of urinary masses, while the most common genital masses are hydrometrocolpos and ovarian cysts (Fig 6–3). Malignant abdominal masses are uncommon in this age group (although neuroblastoma occurs rarely), but pelvic masses with malignant potential (e.g., sacrococcygeal teratoma) do occur.

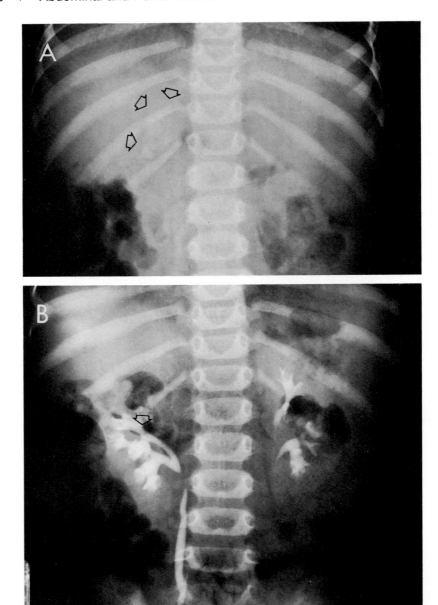

Fig 6–4.—Neuroblastoma. **A,** supine abdominal film of this 2-year-old boy shows a few faint calcifications in the region of the right adrenal gland *(arrows)*. **B,** 5-minute film from the IVU shows the right collecting system displaced inferiorly and laterally *(arrow)*. Note that the calyces are not distorted but displaced. This is a typical finding in neuroblastoma.

ONE MONTH TO TWO YEARS OF AGE

Once again, the urinary masses predominate, with Wilms' tumor and hydrone-phrosis occurring with equal frequency. Nonrenal retroperitoneal masses such as neuroblastoma now become more common (Fig 6–4). The gastrointestinal mass of most concern now becomes the intussusception (see Fig 4–24).

OLDER THAN TWO YEARS

Once a child reaches 2 years of age, the incidence of genitourinary system mass become less, and the differential diagnoses broaden. Traumatic lesions, inflamma-tory processes (e.g., from a perforated appendix), and the more unusual hepatic lesions are now considered (see Fig 5–3). However, Wilms' tumor and neuroblas-toma remain high in the differential diagnoses. The lymphomatous masses in the abdomen become a strong consideration in the older age group.

LOCATION OF THE MASS

After age, the *location* of the mass is the next important consideration. If a neo-nate has a flank mass, the chances are great that it will be a multicystic or hydro-nephrotic kidney. A less likely right upper quadrant mass is a hepatoblastoma. In a 2-year-old, a right upper quadrant mass suggests a neuroblastoma or Wilms' tu-mor. Consider all the normal viscera in locating the center of the mass. This helps form the differential diagnosis.

SYMPTOMS

In many instances when a mass is palpated, either by the parents or a physician, there are no *symptoms*. However, symptoms or signs such as jaundice or profuse

TABLE 6–2.—IMAGING PROCEDURES, BY SIGNS AND SYMPTOMS, IN CHILDREN WITH AN ABDOMINAL-PELVIC MASS

SIGNS OR SYMPTOMS	INITIAL TEST	SECOND TEST (AFTER PLAIN FILMS)	LOOKING FOR
Hypertension	IVU	US	Renal or suprarenal tumor, renal vascular lesion
Jaundice	US	NM	Obstruction of biliary system, choledochal cyst
Fever, right lower quadrant mass	BE*		Appendiceal abscess
Colicky abdominal pain, bloody diarrhea	BE		Intussusception
Projectile vomiting, nonbilious	UGI†		Pyloric stenosis
Hepatic mass	US	NM, CT, angiography	Hepatoblastoma, vascular tumor, resectability
Splenomegaly	US		Patency of portal vein, liver pathology, portal hypertension, masses of spleen

*If diagnosis of acute appendicitis is made clinically, no imaging procedure is necessary; if chronic or atypical, may do BE to show mass effect.
†When pyloric tumor ("olive") is felt, no imaging procedure is needed.

diarrhea provide clues. A jaundiced patient with a right upper quadrant mass may have a choledochal cyst, while the child with a flank mass and profuse secretory diarrhea may have a catecholamine-secreting neuroblastoma.

Specific attention should be paid to symptoms in children with pelvic masses. Because of the relationship of the pelvic mass to the bladder, bowel, and sacral nerve complex, these children may present with dysfunction of one or more of these systems. Since masses (other than those associated with the ovaries and uterus) occur in the pelvis nearly as frequently as they do in the upper abdominal retroperitoneal areas, any child with bladder, bowel, or neurologic symptoms should be suspected of having a pelvic mass; and the diagnostic work-up—appropriate history, physical examination and imaging procedures (Table 6–2)—should proceed accordingly.

IMAGING PRINCIPLES

Many of these principles have been discussed previously. For newborns, ultrasound is generally the first test because most masses are of genitourinary origin (multicystic kidney, hydronephrosis), and most of them are cystic with characteristic ultrasonic appearance. Since a better intravenous urogram can be obtained after a child is a week or two old, this procedure can be done later.

Once the presence of a mass is firmly established and its site determined, the extent of the lesion should be defined (Table 6–3). Computerized tomography has been the most precise imaging method to define the intra-abdominal extent of a tumor.

SPECIFIC LESIONS

NEOPLASMS

The most common abdominal or pelvic tumors of childhood are Wilms' tumor and neuroblastoma.

WILMS' TUMOR

This is an intrarenal tumor (Fig 6–5) with peak incidence between 2 and 5 years of age. Although the presenting symptom is frequently an abdominal flank mass, the tumor is associated with hematuria in 20% of patients. It is commonly asymptomatic, but occasionally fever and pain are symptoms. Hypertension may be present.

TABLE 6–3.—IMAGING WORK-UP IN PATIENTS WITH ASYMPTOMATIC*
ABDOMINAL MASSES

AGE	INITIAL TEST AFTER PLAIN FILM	REASON
Neonate	US	Localizes mass; easily discriminates solid from cystic lesions
1 month to 2 years	IVU or US	Localizes lesion. Total body opacification phase, then US and/or CT, depending on findings
>2 years	Cannot set guidelines. Determined by history and physical examination	Variable

*If symptomatic, go to most appropriate diagnostic test for the probable disease.

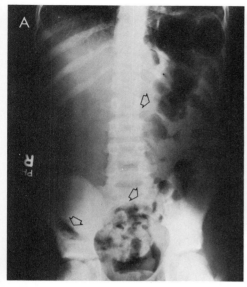
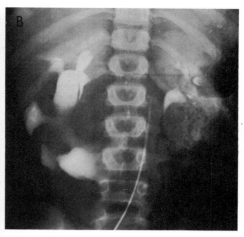

Fig 6–5.—Wilms' tumor. **A,** abdominal film of this 4-year-old boy shows a right-sided abdominal mass displacing bowel inferiorly and to the left *(arrows).* **B,** 5-minute film from the IVU shows a markedly distorted right kidney. Note that the calyces are hydronephrotic and distorted. This is typical for an intrarenal tumor, most commonly a Wilms' tumor.

The radiographic findings are those of distortion of the internal renal architecture. Infrequently, the tumor is large enough to completely obstruct and shut down the kidney. It is uncommon to see calcification. In general, the prognosis is good but depends almost entirely on the histologic type (favorable vs. unfavorable) and staging of the lesion.

For the work-up of a child with an abdominal mass, see Table 6–2. However, once the primary diagnosis is made, the extent of the tumor should be evaluated on the basis of natural history of tumor spread and sites of common metastases. With Wilms' tumor, it is crucial that the inferior vena cava be evaluated, as the tumor often grows directly into the renal veins, the inferior vena cava, and occasionally the heart. Knowledge of tumor in this region will determine if a thoracoabdominal exploration is necessary. The vena cava is best and least invasively evaluated by real-time ultrasound.

Evaluation of the chest—a common site of tumor metastasis—is best done by CT examination. Thus, once the primary lesion and site are known, specific evaluations can be undertaken.

NEUROBLASTOMA

This is a lesion of the sympathetic nerve chain and may arise anywhere along the axis of these sympathetic nerves (see Fig 6–4).

About half of these tumors arise in the abdomen and appear most frequently in the adrenal gland—the suprarenal region. The majority of neuroblastomas occur in children aged 6 months to 5 years. Unlike the asymptomatic presentation of a child with Wilms' tumor, many children with neuroblastoma present with weight loss, irritability, fever, and anemia. A few show excessive catecholamine production and have such symptoms as skin flushing, perspiration, diarrhea, and/or headaches. On physical examination, there may well be hypertension and tachypnea.

The plain-film findings frequently show stippled calcification, with lateral and downward displacement of the kidney. Neuroblastoma has a rather poor prognosis if the child is over 1 year of age. By the time it is diagnosed, it has frequently metastasized to the skeleton, as well as to the bone marrow and the liver.

After the primary neuroblastoma is discovered, evaluation of the bones and the liver is necessary. Liver metastases can be shown by computerized tomographic and radionuclide studies, while radiographs and/or radionuclide studies are best for bone lesions.

HEPATIC TUMORS

These lesions are certainly less common than either Wilms' tumor or neuroblastoma. They are presented here because their imaging evaluation is complex and demands the use of multiple procedures. The two malignant liver tumors seen most frequently are hepatoblastoma and hepatocellular carcinoma. The more common benign hepatic lesions are vascular, such as the hemangioendothelioma. Children with these tumors come to the physician with complaints either of a mass in the upper abdomen or enlargement of the abdomen. Liver dysfunction with jaundice and ascites is less frequently seen.

The initial imaging procedure, after the plain film, is an ultrasound of the right upper quadrant to define the site of abnormality. Because, in most instances, the surgeon would like to know about the resectability of the lesion, the studies that best demonstrate anatomical detail are performed next. These include computed tomography and angiography (see Chap. 9). The degree of functional impairment, as well as the extent of the lesion, is elucidated by radionuclide study.

This, then, is quite different from the evaluation for Wilms' tumor or neuroblastoma. Knowledge of the natural history of the disease, as well as the necessity for precise anatomical detail for surgical resection, demands an extensive multimodality preoperative work-up.

LYMPHOMA

Hodgkin's and non-Hodgkin's lymphomas are frequent malignancies of childhood. While most children do not present with an abdominal mass (see Chap. 2), occasionally a palpable abdominal mass *is* the initial presenting sign. The reason for including lymphomas in this discussion is to remind you that lymphomatous infiltration (as well as leukemic infiltration) of the kidneys, liver, and spleen does occur. When evaluating the abdomen for visceromegaly or mass, these diseases should be considered.

RHABDOMYOSARCOMA

This is the most common of the soft tissue sarcomas. In 16% of cases, the tumor originates in the genitourinary system. The vagina, bladder, testicular or paratesticular region, or prostate may be the primary site. It originates from the same embryonic mesenchyma that gives rise to skeletal muscle and is a major diagnostic consideration when you are faced with a solid pelvic mass. It occurs in any age-group, with 10% appearing in the first year of life; these young infants have an especially poor prognosis. The tumor metastasizes via the lymph and the bloodstream; no specific organ system predominates in metastatic spread. Therefore, the radiographic work-up would include evaluation of bone, chest, lymph nodes, etc.

PREGNANCY—THE MOST COMMON PELVIC MASS IN FEMALES

Evaluation of pelvic masses begins, for girls over 9 years of age, with a pregnancy test or an ultrasound study (see Fig 6–2). Careful longitudinal and transverse scans are done to rule out the easily diagnosible intrauterine pregnancy. The pelvic mass is defined, and the diagnostic possibilities may be limited to a select few.

SUGGESTED READING

1. Swischuk L.E.: *Radiology of the Newborn and Young Infant,* ed. 2. Baltimore, Williams & Wilkins Co., 1980 pp. 490–497.
2. Caffey J.: *Pediatric X-ray Diagnosis,* ed. 7. Chicago, Year Book Medical Publishers, Inc., 1978, pp. 1783–1785.
3. Kirks D.R., Merten D.F., Grossman H., Bowie J.D.: Diagnostic imaging of pediatric abdominal masses: An overview. *Pediatr. Clin. North Am.* 19:527, 1981.

CHAPTER 7

The Skeleton

THE SECOND MOST FREQUENT radiographic study (after the chest film) is that of the pediatric skeleton. The most common indication for such studies is, of course, trauma. In order to understand the disease processes that occur in the pediatric age group, one must first know the skeletal anatomy. The skull and spine will be covered in Chapter 8.

ANATOMY

Long Bones

The two physiologic mechanisms of bone production and development are endochondral (long bones) and intramembranous ossification (flat bones). The long bone of a child is divided into four areas (Fig 7–1):
1. the *diaphysis*—the shaft of the long bone,
2. the *metaphysis*—the area of cartilaginous calcification and ossification where the bone flares,
3. the *physis*—the lucent line where growth takes place prior to calcification of the cartilage,
4. the *epiphysis*, or secondary ossification center—a portion of which interfaces with the joint as the articular cartilage and allows movement within the joint.

The center of the long bone is the medullary cavity, while the outer bone is called the cortex. Some long bones (e.g., the femur) have a nonarticulating *apophysis* (see Fig 7–1), which is similar to the epiphysis but does not contribute to the length of the bone (e.g., the greater trochanter). In the growing pediatric skeleton, blood supply is primarily to the metaphysis, and many of the disease processes and roentgen findings are seen in this region. For example, hematogeneous osteomyelitis is visible most often in the metaphysis; and, similarly, metastases travel hematogenously to the metaphysis.

FLAT BONES

In the flat or membranous bones, there is no diaphysis, metaphysis, or physis but, rather, a mesenchymal network or membrane attracts osteoblasts, which form osteoid. Membranous bones include the mandible, parts of the skull, the clavicles, and the sternum. There are equivalent diaphyseal, metaphyseal, and epiphyseal areas, however, which behave very similarly to their counterparts in the appendicular skeleton.

UNIQUE FEATURES

The skeleton of children is quite different from that of adults. The child's bones are obviously still growing, developing, and modeling; therefore, many ossification

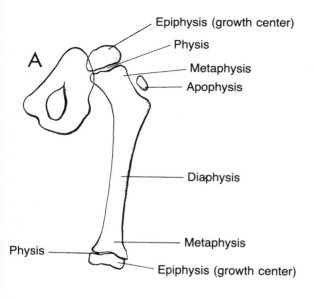

Epiphysis (growth center)
Physis
Metaphysis
Apophysis
Diaphysis
Metaphysis
Physis
Epiphysis (growth center)

Fig 7–1.—A, schematic drawing of a normal femur. **B,** radiograph of a normal femur.

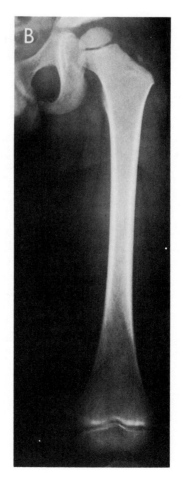

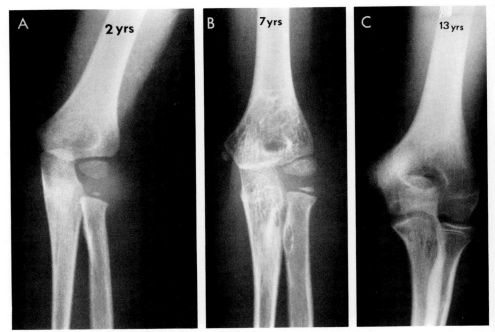

Fig 7–2.—A, B, C, the normal elbow at different stages of development. Note the appearance of the various ossification centers as the child matures.

centers are constantly appearing and fusing with the main skeleton (Fig 7–2). Because these ossification centers may appear fragmented and may ossify in a multicentric fashion, they can easily simulate chip fractures. Therefore, get comparison views if there is any question.

Injuries to the metaphyseal region, physis, and epiphysis are much more damaging in children than in adults because the growth plate is disturbed. These are called Salter-Harris fractures and given a prognostic rating according to the severity of the growth-plate injury (Fig 7–3). Severe length discrepancies and other growth disturbances can occur from fractures in these regions.

Another unique difference between the pediatric and adult skeleton is the low frequency of dislocations (complete disruption of the joints with loss of contact between articulating surfaces) of otherwise normal joints. Because children's capsular and ligamentous structures are two to five times stronger than the weakest part of the growth plate, the growth plate fractures first, and dislocation occurs less frequently.

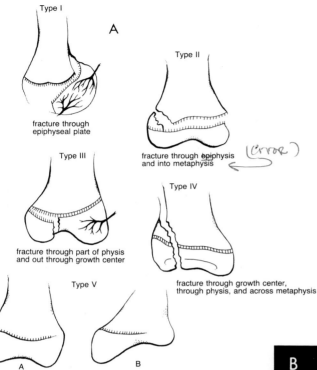

Type I

fracture through
epiphyseal plate

Type II

fracture through epiphysis (Error)
and into metaphysis

Type III

fracture through part of physis
and out through growth center

Type IV

fracture through growth center,
through physis, and across metaphysis

Type V

A   B

crush injury to physis

Fig 7–3.—A, Salter-Harris classification of fractures
involving the growth plate. Prognosis depends on
integrity of the blood supply and fracture type. Salter IV
and V have a worse prognosis than I, II, and III. B,
proximal phalange shows a typical Salter II fracture. The
fracture line extends through the physis and into the
metaphysis.

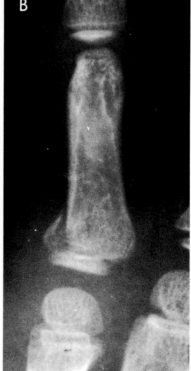

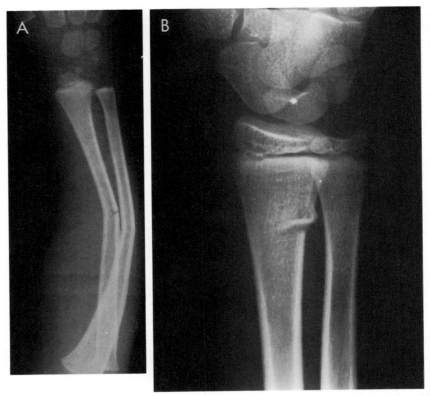

Fig 7–4.—A, greenstick fracture. The fracture extends halfway through the diaphysis, while the other cortex remains intact. **B,** torus fracture. Note the buckling at the medial aspect of the distal radius, while the lateral border remains intact.

The growing bones of children are also unique in that they are more "plastic" and more likely to bend before they fracture (Fig 7–4). Because of this resiliency, children are more likely to have incomplete fractures, two of which have characteristic names—the *greenstick* fracture and the *torus* fracture. The greenstick fracture is characterized by a bowed long bone with a break on the convex surface but complete cortical continuity on the concave surface. In the torus fracture, there is buckling on only one side of the cortex (see Fig 7–4).

In children, the periosteum is constantly growing. Therefore, it is less firmly attached to the diaphysis, or shaft, of the long bone and is more likely to tear and thus be elevated by trauma and hematoma formation. The periosteum reacts by laying down a thick layer of new bone. In contrast, the periosteum at the ends of the long bones is not loosely attached but rather firmly adherent to the metaphyseal regions. Twisting injuries here cause avulsion of a piece of bone from the metaphysis. This type of "bucket-handle" injury or avulsion "corner fracture" is commonly found in cases of child abuse (discussed below) (Fig 7–5).

We can estimate bone maturation by comparing radiographs of the wrists and hands with those in an atlas by Greulich and Pyle.[1] They also provide standard deviations in normal children.

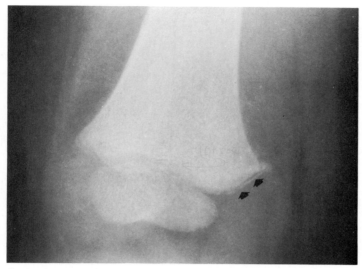

Fig 7–5.—Bucket-handle fracture of distal femur. A thin avulsion of bone at the femoral metaphysis *(arrows)* resembles the resting handle of a bucket. This fracture is commonly seen in the battered child syndrome.

THE GENERAL APPROACH

Before diagnosing specific bony abnormalities, it is important to evaluate the film as a whole. Is the film overexposed? You can judge by looking at the soft tissues and seeing whether they are "burnt out" or clearly visible. If you cannot see them easily, the film is overexposed. If the bones are so light that the trabecular pattern is indistinct or invisible, the film is underexposed. The overexposed film can sometimes be salvaged by viewing in front of a high-intensity illuminator. The underexposed film is ideal for examining soft tissues but not much else.

It is also important to look at any bony abnormality in two or more views. Fractures are easily missed if one relies on just a single view of the area. Comparison views are frequently necessary.

We use the *ABCS* system (from Forrester, Brown, and Nesson's *Radiology of Joint Diseases*)[3] to evaluate the bones:

A = alignment
B = bone size, shape, texture, mineralization, and maturation
C = cartilage and joint space
S = soft tissue

We will discuss the components of the ABCS system in reverse order:

S—Soft tissues (including "fat pads").—As in other areas of the body, the soft tissues give clues to the site and kind of injury (Table 7–1; Fig 7–6).

C—Cartilage and joint space.—Remember, we don't see the joint space alone. Rather, we see the noncalcified articular cartilage and joint space (Fig 7–7). Since only a small portion of this region is joint space, any narrowing may well be significant. The "joint space" should be symmetric and smooth without any calcifications or disruptions (see Fig 7–7).

TABLE 7–1.—ABNORMALITIES OF SOFT TISSUE*

WHAT TO LOOK FOR	DISEASE
Soft tissue swelling	Most likely site of bone abnormality, hemorrhage, traumatic edema, inflammation, neoplastic abnormality
"Fat-pad" elevation	Fluid within a joint displacing the periarticular fat
Muscle wasting	Disuse, neuromuscular abnormality, chronic disease of any etiology requiring lots of bed rest
Calcifications	Old trauma; hemangiomas; metabolic, parasitic, or connective tissue disorders (dermatomyositis, scleroderma)
Opaque foreign bodies	Glass (specifically leaded glass, such as pop bottles) is often visible on a radiograph
Gas in tissue planes	Penetrating trauma, infection by gas-forming bacteria
Adjacent surprises	Unsuspected renal or appendiceal calculi, especially on lumbar spine films

*Modified from Troupin R.H.: *Diagnostic Radiology in Clinical Medicine*, ed. 2. Chicago, Year Book Medical Publishers, Inc., 1978, p. 54.

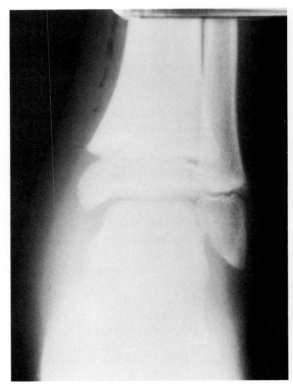

Fig 7–6.—Soft tissue swelling. Note the swelling of the left medial malleolus. Did you note the air in the soft tissues at the upper margin of the film? This swelling was due to a puncture wound that subsequently became infected with gas-forming organisms.

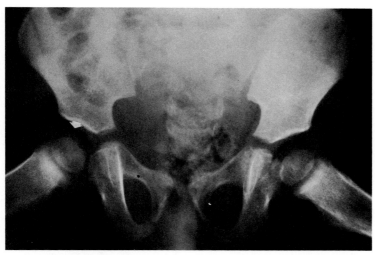

Fig 7–7.—Vacuum phenomenon. The arrow points to a lucent (black) line outlining the cartilaginous head of the femur. This lucency, often seen in the large joints of children, is caused by pulling, resulting in a vacuum in the joint that allows nitrogen to enter and outline the articular cartilage of the bone.

B—Bone size, shape, texture, mineralization, and maturation.—The configuration of the bone and its special relationship helps determine the presence of fractures, dislocations, or congenital anomalies. By looking at the bone surface—the cortex—you can detect pathophysiologic abnormalities. With the exception of so-called physiologic periosteal new bone deposition on the diaphysis of infantile bones, all other periosteal changes, particularly if asymmetric, should be regarded as abnormal. Remember, periosteum is *normally not visible.* It is only seen when it has been stimulated to lay down new bone, or the bone beneath it has been resorbed. With an osteomyelitic process, you can see cortical destruction along with reparative periosteal new bone (Fig 7–8).

REED'S RULE #14—*The periosteum is* not *normally seen.*

Next, we look at the texture of the new bone with its normally uniform trabecular pattern and uniform mineralization. We diagnose metastatic disease and infection by the permeative destructive nature of bone involvement (Fig 7–9). These lesions have no well-defined margins. At this time, we can also detect metabolic disorders such as rickets and scurvy (Fig 7–10).

Bone maturation (see above) becomes important when suspecting certain diseases such as hypothyroidism, where the bone age is markedly decreased.

A—Alignment of bones.—Disruption of bone cortex and articular surfaces is easy to spot when you look for it!!

REED'S RULE #15—*When viewing an extremity, try to imagine the appearance of the patient. An excellent example is bowed legs or knock knees.*

In order to make an intelligent decision about the radiograph of a child's bones,

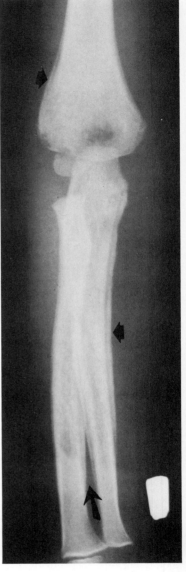

Fig 7–8.—Osteomyelitis. The ulna, radius, and humerus all exhibit a smooth periosteal reaction *(arrows).* The radius has a lytic defect at its distal third. This child has sickle cell disease with multifocal osteomyelitis.

the radiologist must know a few important clinical facts, such as the patient's age, sex, race, prior treatment, and whether this is a generalized or local bone disturbance.

Age.—As discussed in the work-up of a child with an abdominal mass, the occurrence of lesions at different ages helps to form the differential diagnosis. For example, a 6-year-old is more likely to have aseptic necrosis of the capital femoral epiphysis (Legg-Calvé-Perthes disease), while hip disease in a teenager is often a slipped capital femoral epiphysis.

Sex.—Hemophilia affects males; therefore, it follows that arthropathy and bone changes are found only in males.

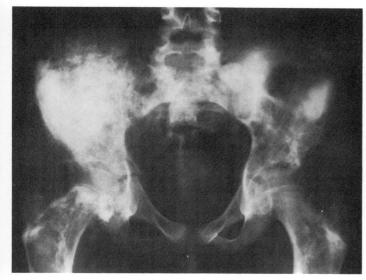

Fig 7–9.—Metastasis. Careful attention to the texture of the bone will show areas of lucency *(black)* and sclerosis *(white).* These correspond to lytic and blastic lesions caused by a medulloblastoma that metastasized to bone. While lytic metastases are commonly seen, blastic ones are quite infrequent.

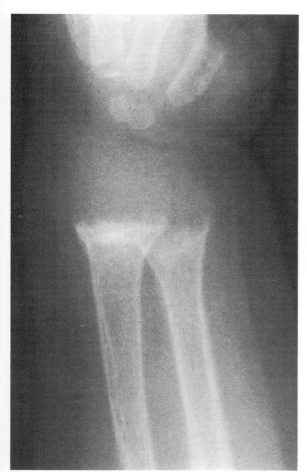

Fig 7–10.—Rickets. The bones appear washed out, and the metaphyses are indistinct and appear "frayed." They also flare at the ends, giving a cupped appearance. Cupping and fraying are typical of rickets.

Race.—Sickle cell anemia, Gaucher's disease, and thalassemia are important considerations in different racial and ethnic backgrounds—sickle cell disease in blacks, Gaucher's in Jewish children, and thalassemia in children of Mediterranean ancestry.

Prior treatment.—It is important for the radiologist to know whether the lesion has been partially treated, since it may display a much different roentgenographic appearance in the treated state. For example, a healing or treated bone cyst appears much different than the untreated variety.

Generalized or local disease.—Finally, the radiologist must know whether this is the only bone involved or whether the disease affects multiple bones. Histiocytosis, fibrous dysplasia, and metastases are multiple bone diseases, while simple bone cysts and Brodie's abscess are most commonly isolated disorders (see Fig 7–9). Therefore, a skeletal survey or bone scan frequently is helpful.

COMMON PEDIATRIC PROBLEMS

TRAUMA

Since trauma is the most frequent indication for skeletal examinations, it is important to know the normal variants that may appear (see Fig 7–2). An excellent source of normal variants is found in the books of Keats[4] and Kohler.[5] It is important to compare sides when one is in doubt about the presence of a fracture (Fig 7–11).

Let's start by looking at the fetus, which is rarely traumatized because it is in a protected environment—an amniotic fluid "water bath." Fractures, however, may occur in congenital diseases such as osteogenesis imperfecta. This disease is characterized by multiple partial and complete fractures in many bones (Fig 7–12).

During difficult deliveries, such as breech presentations, fractures may be sustained; the most common ones involve the clavicles and skull. Since the infant is

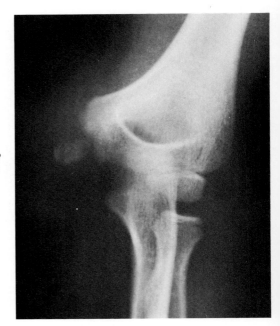

Fig 7–11.—Do you see the abnormality? (See Appendix 2.) Compare this elbow with those in Figure 7–2.

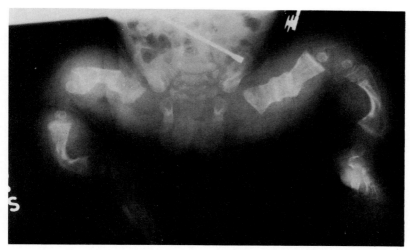

Fig 7–12.—Osteogenesis imperfecta. This newborn (the umbilical clamp is still in place) shows bowed and fractured lower extremities. Note the "crinkling" of the left femur. These fractures occurred in utero and resulted from unusually fragile bones due to a congenital defect in collagen architecture.

not very mobile during the first year of life, most injuries and fractures are secondary to various kinds of accidents. Particular findings, however, lead the radiologist to suspect child abuse—the battered child syndrome. These include multiple fractures in different stages of healing (indicating different times of occurrence), metaphyseal corner ("bucket-handle") fractures (Figs 7–5, 7–13,A), and, particularly, posterior rib fractures (Fig 7–13,B).

One must not, however, confuse the normal appositional new bone formation in infants from 2 to 6 months of age with pathologic periosteal elevation. Rather, this is, as previously stated, normal periosteal bone deposition. It is bilaterally symmetric and found in the humeri, femora, and tibiae. These are not fractures, nor do they denote any trauma (Fig 7–14).

When it is necessary to determine the age of a fracture, remember the younger the child, the faster the healing. In all children, however, the initial reparative process—periosteal reaction—begins 7 to 14 days after the original injury.

We have found the following "trauma tips"—factors unique to pediatrics—useful to keep in mind during the reading of children's radiographs.

1. The clavicle is prone to greenstick fractures, which may be hard to visualize. One must take films in at least three views to make sure the child does not have a fracture.
2. The elbow has so many secondary ossification centers that it is imperative to view the opposite elbow for comparison (see Fig 7–11).
3. The *supermarket elbow* usually results from a sudden pull on a child's arm as the mother is rushing through her shopping. If the radius is dislocated, the child will not move the arm (Fig 7–15). The radius must be in direct relationship to the capitulum, regardless of the position of the elbow. The fat-pad sign is an especially valuable clue in trauma (Fig 7–16).
4. Stress fractures, although unusual, may occur in the proximal tibia, usually following extreme exercise (Fig 7–17).

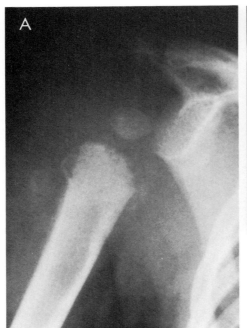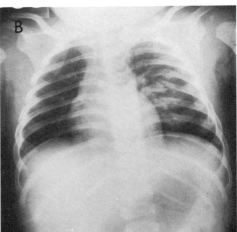

Fig 7–13.—A, a bucket-handle fracture of the right humerus. (see Fig 7–5). **B,** can you find all the abnormalities in this battered child? (See Appendix 2.)

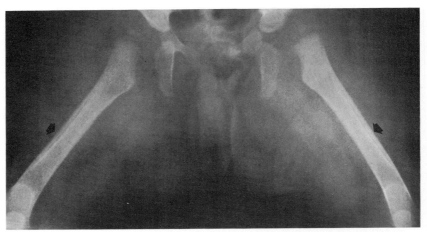

Fig 7–14.—Appositional new bone formation. This frontal view of a 2-month-old child shows what could be mistaken for periosteal reaction on both lateral aspects *(arrows)*. This normal variant can be present up to 6 months of age and reflects rapid bone growth rather than a disease state.

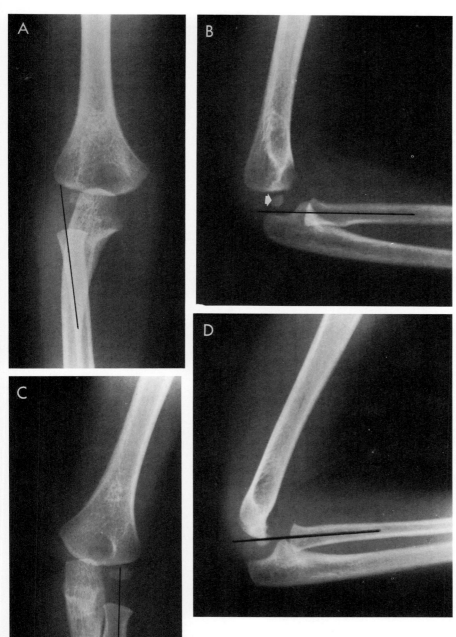

Fig 7–15.—"Nursemaid" or "supermarket" elbow. **A, B,** a line drawn through the shaft of the radius shows that the radius does not articulate with the capitulum *(arrow).* This dislocation is caused by a sharp pulling motion, caused in the old days by a nursemaid and in more modern times by a mother or guardian pulling a child. It often occurs in the supermarket; hence the name. **C, D,** normal realignment.

Fig 7–16.—Positive fat pad sign. While the fracture is not visible, the posterior fat pad is displaced so that it is now visible *(arrows)*. This is an indirect sign of trauma and reflects joint effusion.

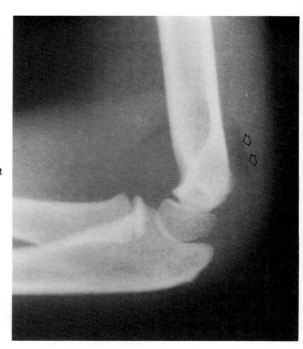

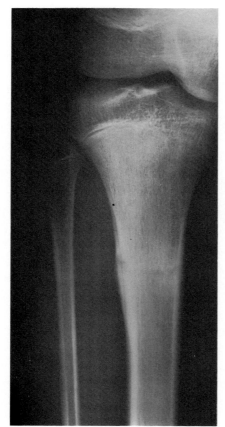

Fig 7–17.—Stress fracture. The tibia shows a zone of sclerosis along the midshaft and periosteal reaction as well.

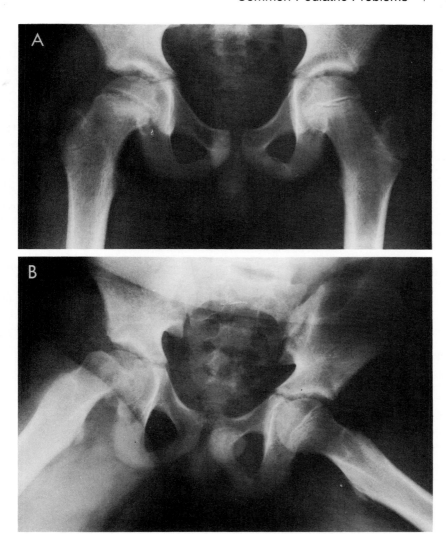

Fig 7–18.—Slipped capital femoral epiphysis. **A,** this film of the hip was taken in neutral position and shows asymmetry in the physis of the femoral heads. The right appears wider, and the head appears somewhat medially displaced. In all suspected cases of slipped capital femoral epiphyses, a frog-leg lateral film is taken **(B)**. **B,** frog-leg lateral film shows complete separation of the right femoral head. This will require pinning of the head to the neck.

5. A toddler's fracture, seen in children between the ages of 9 months and 3 years, is an oblique, nondisplaced fracture of the distal tibial shaft.
6. The slipped capital femoral epiphysis is a Salter I fracture of the femoral head (Fig 7–18). This injury is found in adolescents, and there is a significant incidence of bilaterality.
7. Metaphyseal corner fractures, multiple injuries, and, particularly, posterior rib fractures, are clues to child abuse (see Fig 7–13).

OSTEOMYELITIS

Osteomyelitis is usually acquired via hematogenous spread of organisms to the bone. Since the greatest blood supply is in the metaphysis, this region has a predilection for osteomyelitis. A small focus of these purulent organisms causes abscess formation in the marrow with an increase in local pressure, followed by local deossification and destruction of the cortex (Fig 7–19,A and B). The epiphysis is usually spared because of the tight adherence of the periosteum to the metaphysis. However, the shaft of the bone is readily permeable to infection because the periosteum is loosely adherent, and organisms may ascend the shaft of the bone or the medullary cavity.

Deep puncture wounds may also cause osteomyelitis in children. One of the more common organisms introduced via a puncture wound is *Pseudomonas*, while staphylococcal osteomyelitis is most common in hematogenously spread disease (see Fig 7–8).

The clinical symptoms precede the radiographic findings by 7 to 14 days. For this reason, a radioisotope study is frequently more helpful in the early diagnosis of acute osteomyelitis.

If the diagnosis is made promptly and treatment is successful, healing usually occurs without significant growth disturbance. However, prolonged infection prior to the diagnosis or severe involvement of a joint—septic arthritis—can have long-term sequelae (Fig 7–19,C).

The radiographic findings of acute, healing, and chronic osteomyelitis are summarized below.

Acute Osteomyelitis (0–2 weeks)
   Soft tissue swelling initially
   Loss of cortical margin
   Focal demineralization of bone
   Faint periosteal new bone formation (7–14 days after onset)
Healing Phase (2–4 weeks)
   Destroyed bone with irregular areas of sclerosis and lysis
   Sequestrum—dense devascularized bone fragment within an area of pus and
      granulation tissue
   Involucrum—peripheral shell of supporting bone laid down by the periosteum
      around the old disease
Chronic Osteomyelitis (either unusual localized osteomyelitis or improperly
   treated)
   Diffuse bone production with little or no destruction
   Occasional draining sinus or lucent area in the midst of the sclerotic bone

Certain children, however, are at high risk for osteomyelitis and its complications. These include neonates who have a high incidence of both β-streptococcal osteomyelitis and septic arthritis. Sickle cell patients have a high incidence of *Salmonella* osteomyelitis, which is frequently multifocal. However, sickle cell patients with bone infections more often have staphylococcal osteomyelitis. Children with immune deficiencies such as chronic granulomatous disease and agammaglobulinemia are prone to multifocal osteomyelitis or osteomyelitis in unusual areas such as the iliac bones; this is frequently due to unusual organisms.

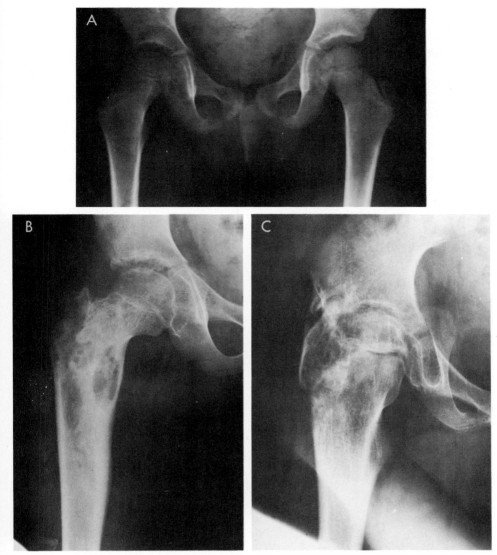

Fig 7–19.—Osteomyelitis. **A,** careful study of both femurs shows that one appears more osteoporotic (blacker) than the other. This was the first sign of abnormality in the right femur. **B,** 4 weeks later. The periosteal reaction and extensive bone destruction are now obvious. **C,** 6 months later. There is ankylosis (fusion of the right hip). Hopefully, this amount of destruction and joint complication will not result if patients receive timely treatment. Early recognition and early treatment prevent such serious sequelae.

METABOLIC DISORDERS

The growing skeleton is susceptible to many nutritional deficiencies and reflects the adequacy of the homeostatic mechanisms (GI tract, liver, kidneys) for handling calcium. Two of the more common disturbances in this category are rickets and hyperparathyroidism, which is usually secondary to chronic renal disease.

Rickets.—In rickets there is a deficiency of vitamin D and, therefore, poorly mineralized osteoid tissue. The trabeculae are fuzzy and irregular and certainly not as distinct as those in normal bone. The metaphyseal regions are irregular, with cupped and frayed metaphyses (see Fig 7–10). The apparent space between the metaphysis and the ossification center is greater than normal, as there is an abundance of uncalcified cartilage. Despite all our advances, the most common cause of rickets in the world today is still nutritional vitamin D deficiency. However, in most medical centers, the most common cause of "rickets" is chronic renal disease. Children with liver disease also may manifest rachitic changes.

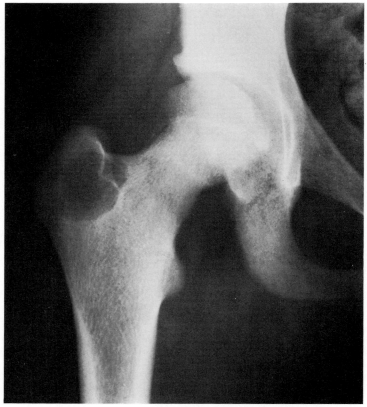

Fig 7–20.—Hyperparathyroidism. This femur shows the radiographic signs of hyperparathyroidism. The cortical margins of the neck (both medial and lateral) of the femur are not visible due to bone resorption. (Compare to neck or femur in Fig 7–1.) Also note the lytic lesion in the greater trochanter. This brown tumor is the result of intraosseous hemorrhage and has all the characteristics of a benign bone lesion. A sclerotic border and the clear zone of demarcation are evidence of its benignity.

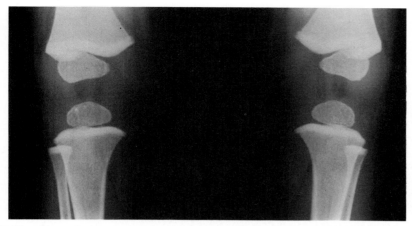

Fig 7–21.—The metaphyses of all the bones, especially the fibula, are sclerotic. This is typical of heavy-metal ingestion. While the femur, tibia, and humerus often have equivocal density in the metaphyses, the ulna and fibula should not be dense at all. Consequently, any metaphyseal density noted in the latter two bones should raise the suspicion of heavy-metal intoxication.

Hyperparathyroidism.—In this disorder, bone resorption far exceeds bone proliferation (osteoclasis far exceeds osteoblastic activity); and, as a result, the bone is resorbed. Radiographically, one sees subperiosteal bone resorption most often along the diaphyses of the phalanges, at the distal clavicles, and along the lamina dura of the teeth. Diffuse demineralization and focal lucent lesions (brown tumors) are other signs of this disorder (Fig 7–20). In chronic renal disease, calcium loss through the urinary system is usually so great that the parathyroids must draw calcium into the blood system from the existing stores in bones to maintain a normal calcium-phosphorous ratio.

Lead intoxication.—Increased calcification of cartilage causes increased density in the metaphyseal regions. This phenomenon is caused by heavy-metal (e.g., lead or bismuth) intoxication. The density is found in both large, weight-bearing bones as well as smaller ones (e.g., tibia and fibula) and in other areas where longitudinal bone growth is occurring most rapidly (Fig 7–21).

BONE TUMORS

Malignant bone tumors are not common in children, but benign bone lesions are frequently seen. Some of the common benign and malignant lesions are described below.

BENIGN LESIONS

Simple bone cyst—a lucent defect at the end of the long bone near the epiphyseal line, most often found in the humerus, femur, or tibia.

Fibrous cortical defect—a well-circumscribed, elliptical lucent lesion in the cortex at the end of a long bone, particularly the femur or tibia. The larger ones are called nonossifying fibromas.

Osteochondroma—a protruberant growth of bone from the diaphysis that has contiguous cortical margins.

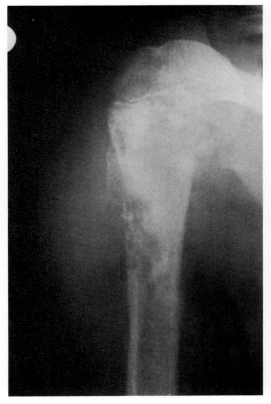

Fig 7–22.—Osteogenic sarcoma. This radiograph displays many of the findings of a malignant bone lesion. The disordered periosteal reaction both medially and laterally and the extensive bone destruction without a clear zone of demarcation between normal and abnormal suggest malignancy.

Enchondroma—a cartilaginous, cystlike lesion often seen in the phalanges and ribs.

Osteoid osteoma—a sclerotic lesion with a central lucent nidus. It occurs in many places, including the long bones and spine.

MALIGNANT LESIONS (Fig 7–22)

Osteogenic sarcoma—occurs mostly during adolescence, frequently in the long bones. This is the most common primary malignant tumor in the pediatric age group, and it is metaphyseal and bone-producing.

Ewing's sarcoma—the second most common tumor in the pediatric age group; it is more common than osteogenic sarcoma under 10 years of age. This lesion may occur in any bone in the mid-diaphyseal region and permeate with a large, soft tissue component. It is frequently found in flat bones, such as those of the pelvis.

Systemic malignancies of bone—leukemia, neuroblastoma (metastatic), retinoblastoma (metastatic), hepatoblastoma (metastatic). These lesions all appear as permeative bone lesions and cannot be *specifically* diagnosed by x-ray.

The radiologist must decide whether the lesion is benign or malignant. Clear signs of a benign lesion include sharp demarcation between the lesion and the normal bone, a sclerotic margin around the lesion, and a nonaggressive pattern of growth. The characteristics most often associated with a malignancy include an accompanying soft tissue mass, an indistinct zone between the normal and abnormal bone—an indistinct zone of demarcation—and permeative, destructive changes in the bone (see Fig 7–22). Remember, however, histologic diagnoses can only be guessed at. Only a biopsy can result in a sure diagnosis (and, at times, even the biopsy may not be correct).

THE ARTHRITIDES

The most common cause for joint swelling in pediatrics is trauma. Usually the history is obtained, and the injury is short-lived. The second most common cause

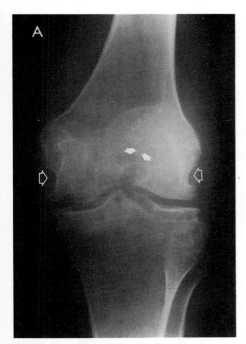

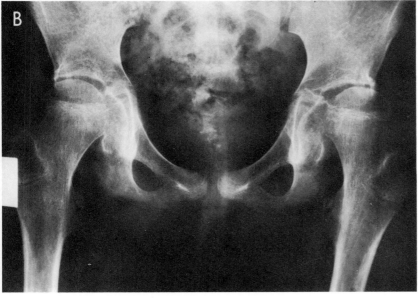

Fig 7–23.—Arthritides. **A,** hemophilia. Hemophilic arthropathy can be recognized by the squaring of the ends of the long bones (compare the distal femur to that in Fig 7–1) and the erosive defects along the condyles *(arrows)*. The joint space narrowing and erosions (the intracondylar notch is also eroded [*arrowheads*]) are typical of arthritis. **B,** juvenile rheumatoid arthritis. Note the joint space narrowing in both hip joints. Osteoporosis is the hallmark of this disease. The left hip is laterally displaced by the synovial proliferation.

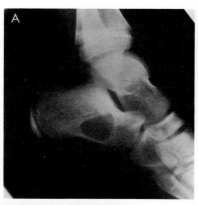

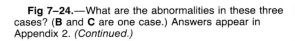

Fig 7–24.—What are the abnormalities in these three cases? (**B** and **C** are one case.) Answers appear in Appendix 2. *(Continued.)*

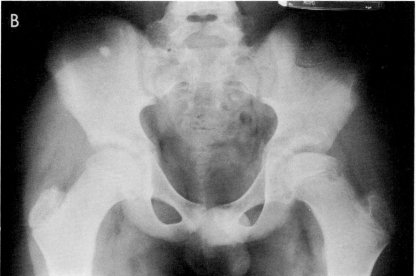

of "arthritis" is infectious—the septic joint. The common organisms in childhood are *Hemophilus influenzae*, *Staphylococcus*, and *Streptococcus*, but the ubiquitous gonococcus cannot be forgotten. Here again, radiographic signs of bone involvement may not be present, but there is joint effusion and swelling. Appropriate clinical maneuvers such as tapping the joint are diagnostic. Less commonly, hemophilic arthritis, rheumatoid arthritis, and arthritides of collagen disease are found (Fig 7–23). What abnormalities do you see in Figure 7–24?

SUGGESTED READING

1. Greulich W.W., Pyle S.I.: *Radiographic Atlas of Skeletal Development of the Hand and Wrist,* ed. 2. Stanford, Calif., Stanford University Press, 1959.
2. Schultz R.J.: *The Language of Fractures.* Baltimore, Williams & Wilkins Co., 1972.
3. Forrester D.M., Brown J.C., Nesson J.W.: *Radiology of Joint Diseases,* ed. 2. Philadelphia, W.B. Saunders Co., 1978.

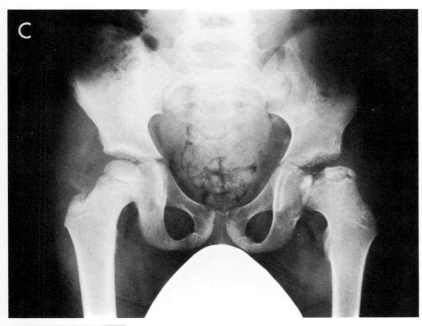

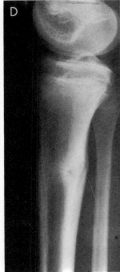

Fig 7–24 (cont.)

4. Keats T.E.: *An Atlas of Normal Roentgen Variants That May Simulate Disease*, ed. 2. Chicago, Year Book Medical Publishers, Inc., 1979.
5. Köhler A.: *Borderlands of the Normal and Early Pathologic in Skeletal Roentgenology*, ed. 10. London, Grune & Stratton, 1956.
6. Ozonoff M.B.: *Pediatric Orthopaedic Radiology*. Philadelphia, W.B. Saunders Co., 1979.

CHAPTER **8**

The Central Nervous System

COMPUTERIZED TOMOGRAPHY has revolutionized the field of neuroradiology. This modality allows for evaluation of the bony calvarium as well as the brain and spinal cord. There remain, however, some good indications for plain-film radiography of the skull and vertebral column.

SKULL AND INTRACRANIAL CONTENTS

ANATOMY

SKULL

The cranial sutures and fontanelles divide the skull into its major bones (Fig 8–1). A suture is a nonossified portion of the membranous bone. (Remember, the majority of the skull is derived from membranous tissue, while the base of the skull and long bones are derived from endochondral ossification.) The metopic and coronal sutures begin at the large, diamond-shaped anterior fontanelle. The midline sagittal suture separates the parietal bones. It extends from the anterior fontanelle to the posterior fontanelle at the posterior aspect of the parietal bones.

The complex occipital bone is composed of six individual bones—two interparietal, one supraoccipital, two extraoccipital, and one basioccipital bone.

The temporal bone, located inferior to the parietal bone and anterior to the occipital bone, includes the mastoid process and structures of the internal ear. The temporal bone extends anteriorly to the sphenoid bone.

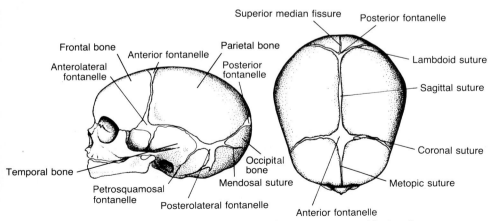

Fig 8–1.—The infant calvarium with major bones, sutures, and fontanelles.

169

The sphenoid bone is the dense structure at the base of the skull and includes the greater and lesser wings and the sella turcica.

The largest bone of the face is the mandible. A routine skull examination should include the mandible, maxilla, orbital structures, and paranasal sinuses (maxillary, ethmoidal, and frontal).

The closure time of various intracranial sutures and fontanelles, as well as the appearance of the paranasal sinuses, is summarized below.

Closure of fontanelles (average range/total range)
    Anterior: 15–18 months/9–24 months
    Posterior: 1–2 months/birth–3 months
Closure of sutures*
    Mendosal: several weeks after birth
    Metopic: 2d year (10% persist throughout life)
    Coronal, sagittal, lambdoidal: about age 30
Appearance of paranasal sinuses (great deal of variation)†
    Ethmoid sinuses: rudimentary air cells at birth but usually no air seen radiographically until 3–6 months
    Maxillary sinuses: rudimentary air cells at birth but usually no air seen radiographically until 3–6 months
    Sphenoidal sinuses: 1–3 years
    Frontal sinuses: 4–8 years

Figure 8–2 shows the multiple views necessary to evaluate the various portions of the skull. It is advisable to know these projections so that optimal visualization of particular sections of the calvarium can be obtained. The calvarium changes dramatically with age as the sutures and fontanelles close. Figure 8–3 shows the maturation process of the skull. Many more sutures are seen in the neonate and young infant than in older children.

INTRACRANIAL CONTENTS

Thus far, we have discussed only the bony vault. Another view, the axial, is used in computed tomography to appreciate intracranial contents. The standard CT scan is performed along the horizontal plane, approximately 20 degrees above the orbital-meatal line (Fig 8–4). In addition to the multiple sections in this plane, the radiologist can obtain direct coronal, as well as lateral and sagittal, sections by computerized reconstruction of the data.

In contrast to the sharp demarcation of various bones of the skull, the lobes of the brain merge imperceptibly on CT scan. It is, therefore, essential to recognize the sulci, fissures, cisterna, and ventricles and to correctly identify the anatomical section. A major landmark is the sylvian fissure between the temporal and parietal lobes. Gray and white matter are easily recognized by their density differences.

Finally, in the neonate with an open fontanelle, a third modality—intracranial

---

*Gooding G.A.: Cranial Sutures and Fontanelles, in Newton T.H., Potts, D.C., eds.: *Radiology of the Skull and Brain,* St. Louis, C. V. Mosby Co., 1971.

†Caffey J.: *Pediatric X-ray Diagnosis,* ed. 7. Chicago, Year Book Medical Publishers, Inc., 1978, p. 111.

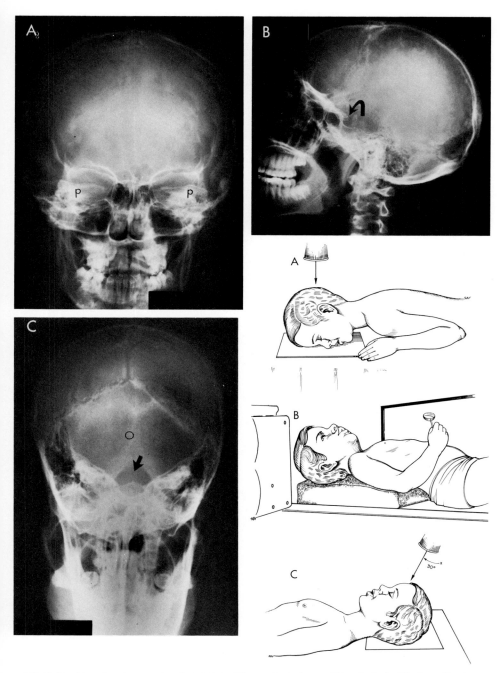

Fig 8–2.—Line drawings and radiographs of the various views of the skull. **A,** PA view. The beam enters the back of the child's head on a line perpendicular to the film, allowing visualization of the petrous pyramids *(p),* which are projected through the orbits. **B,** cross-table lateral view. The beam enters one side of the child's head while the film is on the other. In this way, a horizontal lateral is achieved. This method allows the child to remain comfortable during the procedure, and the entire calvarium as well as the sella turcica *(arrow)* and the cervical spine are nicely displayed. **C,** Towne's view. The beam is directed toward the back of the patient's head at a 30-degree angle. This view is designed to demonstrate the occipital bone *(O)* and the foramen magnum *(arrow).* Basal skull fractures are often seen best in this view.

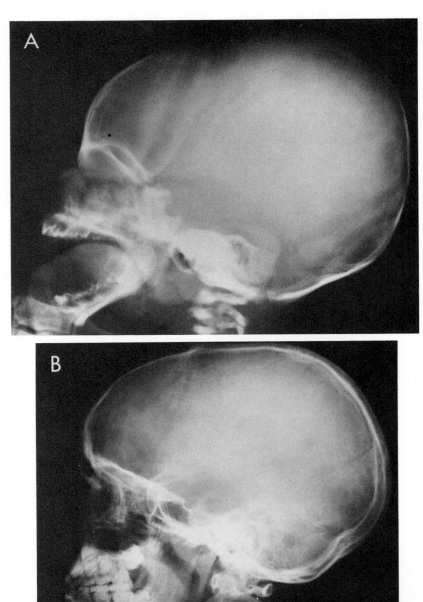

Fig 8–3.—Comparison views of the skull from early childhood through adolescence. Note how the sutures become less obvious and the paranasal sinuses aerate. *(continued)*

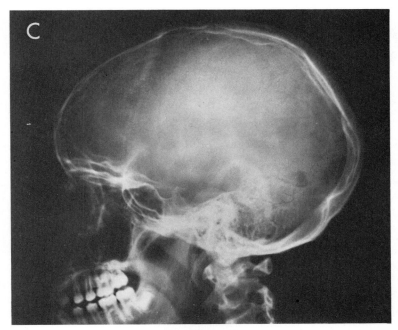

Fig 8–3 (cont.)

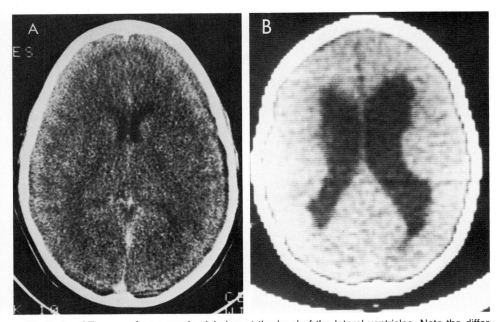

Fig 8–4.—CT scans. **A,** a normal axial view at the level of the lateral ventricles. Note the differentiation between white (black on CT) and gray matter. **B,** a second view, showing the bodies of the lateral ventricles. This child has hydrocephalus, and the CT scan shows dilatation of the ventricles.

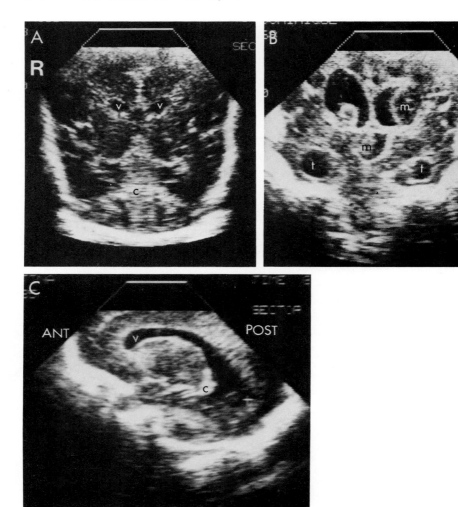

Fig 8–5.—Sonographic evaluation of intracranial contents. **A,** coronal section through the anterior fontanelle. This section is at the level of the frontal horns of the lateral ventricles *(V)*. The caudate nucleus abuts on the lateral aspect of the frontal horns. In premature infants, the immature vascular network on the caudate nucleus is a site of hemorrhage. **B,** Subependymal hemorrhage in a premature infant. The coronal section reveals ventricular dilatation and some asymmetry. There is an echogenic mass *(white m)* in the region of the caudate nucleus. This is the hemorrhage. Blood is in the right frontal horn and in the third ventricle *(black m)*. The temporal horns *(t)* are also dilated. **C,** parasagittal section off the midline reveals the right lateral ventricle *(v)* with a normal choroid plexus *(c)*. The choroid plexus is echogenic and may often be confused with hemorrhage.

ultrasound—can show anatomical detail of the intracranial structures (Fig 8–5). Because of the open fontanelle, sound waves do not have to penetrate the bony calvarium; they easily penetrate the brain and give good anatomical detail, usually demonstrated in both the coronal and sagittal planes.

APPROACH TO THE PLAIN SKULL FILM

Figure 8–2 shows a lateral view of the skull. A systematic approach you can use to examine the skull is to begin from the external surface, work through the calvarium, and down into the face and spine.

THE SOFT TISSUES

Any bulge or enlargement of the soft tissues should be noted. This may be the site of trauma (we suggest looking harder in this region for a fracture) or protuberance of intracranial contents—an encephalocele—or, if at the fontanelle, evidence of increased intracranial pressure.

THE THREE BONY TABLES (Fig 8–6)

THE OUTER TABLE.—This is the extreme bony margin of the skull. Irregularities or disruption of this cortex denote abnormality. Cephalohematoma, osteomyelitis, metastasis, and histiocytosis all affect this portion of the skull (Fig 8–6,A).

THE DIPLOË.—This is the middle table and contains the bone marrow. Severe hemolytic anemia can cause proliferation of bone marrow and enlargement of the diploë, giving a "hair-on-end" appearance (e.g., thalassemia) (Fig 8–6,B).

THE INNER TABLE.—This portion of the bony calvarium is frequently affected by lesions within the cranial vault. The most common "erosion" is normal pacchionian granulation (Fig 8–6,C).

CALVARIUM

Now we are looking through the bone as well as at the generalized bony covering. Pay close attention to the cranial sutures, possible fractures, or intracranial calcifications. While common in adults, "normal calcifications" of the pineal, habenular commissure, choroid plexus, or dura are unusual in childhood (under the age of 15 years).

THE SELLA TURCICA

This is a site commonly affected by increased intracranial pressure. It is also an area affected by one of the more common pediatric tumors—the craniopharyngioma.

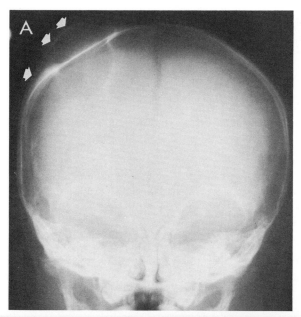

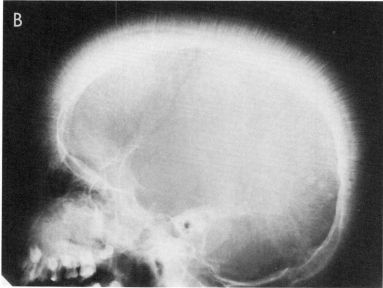

Fig 8–6.—Abnormalities in the tables of the calvarium. **A,** outer table—cephalohematoma. The outer table of the calvarium *(arrows)* is elevated by subperiosteal bleeding. This is a finding during the first days after birth and will eventually heal uneventfully. **B,** diploë or middle table—thalassemia. The extramedullary hematopoiesis that frequently occurs in patients with this disorder expands the diploic region of the calvarium—middle table. The result is a "hair-on-end" appearance, which can be seen in any disorder that results in extramedullary sites for hematopoiesis. **C,** inner table—pacchionian granulation. The inner table *(arrow)* is bowed toward the diploë by rather abundant pacchionian granulation. These are arachnoid extensions that aid with spinal fluid resorption. *(continued)*

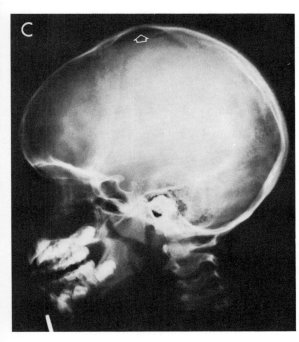

Fig 8–6 (cont.)

THE FACE

The paranasal sinuses, orbits, and nasal structures are easily seen (Fig 8–7). Look for asymmetry, opacification, or bony destruction.

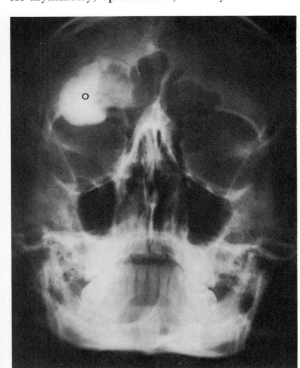

Fig 8–7.—Waters' view of the calvarium. Careful attention to symmetry of the face allows one to detect the large, bony benign tumor *(o)* of the frontal sinus. It is an osteoma.

THE NECK

The soft tissues of the neck and nasopharynx, as well as the cervical spine, are clearly visible. Look for displacement of the air column, mass (this will be a mass effect), or any bony destruction.

On the frontal film (see Fig 8–7), the easiest way to detect an abnormality is to look for asymmetry. The body is, for the most part, symmetric, and a line drawn down the middle of the frontal skull film should result in mirror images of one side of the skull as compared to the other.

INDICATIONS FOR IMAGING EVALUATION

TRAUMA

Over 50% of children with epidural and subdural hematomas do not have changes in the bony skull, i.e., do not have skull fractures.[1] Thus, absence of fracture does not rule out damage to the brain. It is apparent, then, how useful seeing the intracranial contents really is. Similarly, not all children who have head trauma need imaging evaluation. However, the unconscious patient, the child with neurologic findings or changing sensorium, and the patient with a history of severe central nervous system trauma should be evaluated by CT for damage to the intracranial contents. As in all imaging evaluations, the patient should have stable vital signs before being sent for this procedure. Having an intravenous infusion ready and functioning helps the radiologist, as contrast enhancement is frequently necessary. The goal of this evaluation is to detect parenchymal abnormalities or shifts of intracranial contents by either parenchymal or extra-axial lesions and changes in ventricular size and contour.

If a child is brought to the emergency room after trauma and is alert and apparently well *without* a history of unconsciousness, retrograde amnesia, or physical findings suggestive of central nervous system alteration (palpable bony malalignment, CSF discharge from either the ear or nose, ear drum discoloration, absence of neurologic findings), the chances of a fracture or the need for intracranial imaging are extremely small.[2, 3] However, there is still a role for limited and selective use of skull films, especially in cases of possible child abuse or unusual skull fractures. The latter include: (1) *depressed fracture,* where a fragment of bone is pushed in on intracranial contents; (2) *diastatic fracture,* in which the meninges may become entrapped and cause, by the vascular pulsations of CSF, bone erosion and enlargement of the fracture; (3) *fracture through the sinuses;* or (4) *fractures crossing the path of the middle meningeal artery.* If these lesions are seen, CT may be ordered to rule out the complications of these fractures.

One of the indications mentioned above for skull films is that of child abuse. The skull examination is merely the first of a series of skeletal examinations for detecting radiographic evidence of child abuse (see Chap. 7).

When looking for fractures on plain films, remember these rules:
1. Soft tissue swelling often accompanies acute fractures.
2. An acute fracture line is sharp, does not branch, and does not have sclerotic margins.
3. With rare exceptions, there are no sutures within the parietal bone; therefore, any sharp, linear lucency in this region is a fracture until proved otherwise.

4. There are so many vascular grooves and normal variants, it is important to have available one of the standard references for normal skull roentgen variants. (see suggested reading).

Seizures[4]

An imaging procedure is usually not necessary for a child with a febrile seizure. In most instances, the major diagnostic consideration is meningitis, for which a spinal tap is diagnostic. However, the work-up of a child with a nonfebrile seizure is a different matter. Here the major concern is an intracranial mass lesion (tumor, subdural, etc.) causing the seizure. Yet the expectation of finding neurologic changes or abnormalities on plain radiographs or laboratory evaluation (calcium, sodium, magnesium, and glucose) is quite low. One of the best (although nonspecific) tests is the EEG. It detects superficial masses, as well as generalized electrical abnormalities. However, the most sensitive test for detecting a mass lesion is the CT. The efficacy of doing a CT on all nonfebrile seizure patients is certainly questionable. While the yield is extremely small, it may demonstrate a *treatable condition*. The role of CT in nonfebrile seizures will hopefully be clarified in the next several years.

Increased Intracranial Pressure or Enlarging Head Circumference

It is easy to evaluate a child with an open fontanelle for increasing intracranial pressure. The fontanelle bulges when the child is in a sitting position, and the child may also exhibit a high-pitched cry and irritability. Prior to fontanelle closure, ultrasonic evaluation detects ventricular enlargement. Once the fontanelle closes, the sutures may spread before the patient exhibits some of the clinical signs of increased pressure, such as papilledema. Because radiographic signs often precede the clinical clues, you should be familiar with the major radiographic signs of increased intracranial pressure. These are discussed below.

SPREADING OF THE CRANIAL SUTURES.—The coronal suture spreads first but is often difficult to interpret if it is the only finding. It is important to see all of the sutures widened if one is to be sure about increased intracranial pressure. The lateral view is *not* the best view to determine suture spread, as there may be superimposition of right and left sides; rather, the frontal projections—Towne's or PA—are best (Fig 8–8). Children up to the age of 10–12 years (Bell and McCormick[5] say 12 years, while duBoulay[7] says 10) with increased intracranial pressure may have spread sutures before papilledema. Remember that, in neglected or nutritionally starved children, there may be a rebound growth with suture spread as they recover. In this instance, the sutures are spread, but there is no increased intracranial pressure.

ALTERATIONS OF THE SELLA TURCICA.—The cortical outline of the dorsum sellae may become thinned. This leads to eventual erosion of the dorsum, and it becomes truncated and sharpened. Such changes reflect generalized intracranial pressure and are not specific for lesions about the sellae.

Why is there increased intracranial pressure? The differential diagnoses in children include diverse etiologies not considered in adults such as lead encephalopathy, congenitally obstructive hydrocephalus, and congenital arterial-venous malformations such as a vein of Galen aneurysm. Increased intracranial pressure is, of course, a major presenting sign in a child with a brain tumor.

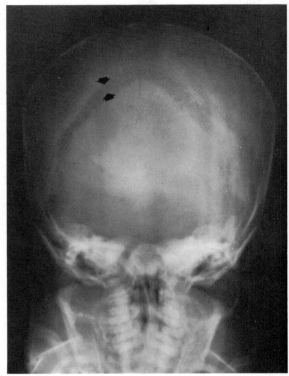

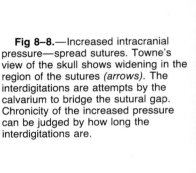

Fig 8–8.—Increased intracranial pressure—spread sutures. Towne's view of the skull shows widening in the region of the sutures *(arrows)*. The interdigitations are attempts by the calvarium to bridge the sutural gap. Chronicity of the increased pressure can be judged by how long the interdigitations are.

CONGENITAL ABNORMALITIES, INCLUDING CONGENITAL INFECTIONS

The neonate with an abnormal configuration of the head should be examined radiographically for premature closure of a suture (craniosynostosis, craniostenosis) (Fig 8–9). We are more concerned about the cranial vault than the intracranial contents. The most common suture to close prematurely is the sagittal suture, giving the patient an elongated head from front to back with a palpable bony ridge over the top (Fig 8–9,A). Radiographically, only a portion of a suture need be closed to result in an abnormal cranial configuration (because functionally the entire suture is closed) (Fig 8–9,B,C).

In the child with an enlarging head, skull films are not specific. In the young infant, ultrasound of the intracranial contents detects congenital anomalies and hydrocephalus, while computerized tomographic studies provide the answer in older children.

The child with a small head may well have one of the congenital infections—the TORCH diseases (TO = toxoplasmosis, R = rubella, C = cytomegalovirus, H = herpes). While gross calcifications are easy to detect on plain skull films, more subtle calcific deposits are best detected on the CT scan.

OTHER INDICATIONS FOR IMAGING EVALUATION OF THE CNS

1. New or progressive neurological findings. CT is very helpful.
2. Work-up of metastatic disease. Both skull films (if this is a primary tumor that commonly goes to bone) and CT (if intracranial metastasis is sought) are indicated.

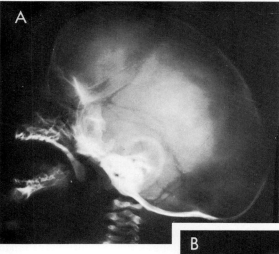

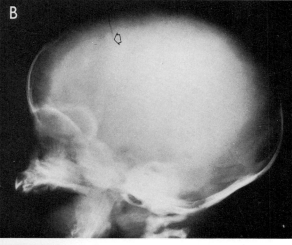

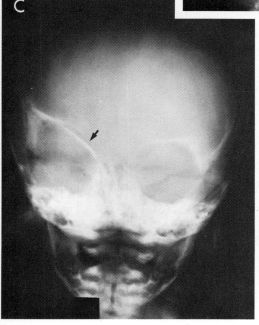

Fig 8–9.—Craniosynostosis (craniostenosis). **A,** this child has a very long head (scaphalocephaly) anteroposteriorly, caused by premature closure of the sagittal suture, which is best seen on a frontal view. The lateral view shows the abnormal head shape. **B,** compare this child to the one in **A.** The head is much shallower due to closure of a part of one coronal suture *(arrow).* **C,** on this frontal film, note the facial asymmetry. The right sphenoid bone (in the right orbit) is elevated because of the premature closure of this coronal suture *(arrow).*

3. Masses of the head and neck such as rhabdomyosarcoma or intraorbital lesions. Both skull radiographs and CT are necessary.

4. Inflammatory sinus disease. Order skull (sinus) films first.

SUPPLEMENTARY PROCEDURES IN EVALUATING THE CENTRAL NERVOUS SYSTEM

ARTERIOGRAPHY

Arteriography is performed by passing a catheter via the femoral artery to the carotid and/or vertebral arteries. The procedure helps map precise arterial anatomy before surgery and is frequently done for tumors to clarify and supplement CT studies.

PNEUMOENCEPHALOGRAPHY AND VENTRICULOGRAPHY

Small volumes of air are introduced into the subarachnoid space via lumbar puncture or into the ventricle via ventricular tap. This defines precise intraventricular and cisternal anatomy so as to detect lesions in, or impinging on, these structures. In general, these studies have been replaced by computerized tomography.

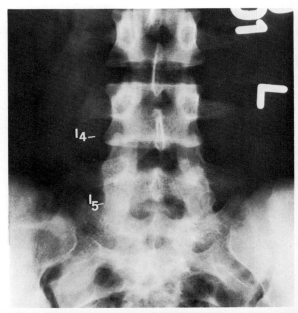

Fig 8–10.—Top, frontal view of the lumbar vertebrae with schematics. L-4 is a normal lumbar vertebra. **Bottom,** schematic diagram explains the various structures and how they contribute to the final product. *A,* vertebral body; *B,* vertebral body plus pedicles in black and spinous process; *C,* superior-inferior articulating facets that have been added; *D,* transverse process. What is wrong with L-5? (See Appendix 2.)

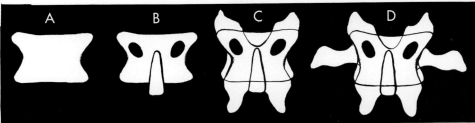

THE SPINE

ANATOMY

The complexities of, and differences among, the cervical, thoracic, lumbar, and sacral segments are beyond the scope of this text; but knowledge of the general configuration of the bony anatomy is crucial (Fig 8–10). The two major views of the spine are the frontal and lateral. It is important to identify (1) the vertebral bodies, (2) the disc spaces between vertebral bodies, (3) the posterior elements, (4) the spinous processes. The vertebral bodies get larger in a cephalic-to-caudal direction. The ring epiphyses are best seen at the corners of the vertebral bodies on the lateral view (Fig 8–11,B).

The alignment of the bony spine is crucial in the radiographic diagnosis of trauma or scoliosis. This is especially true with the cervical spine; a line drawn from C-1 through C-7 along the anterior aspects of the vertebral bodies and a similar line along the posterior aspects, of the vertebral bodies as well as along the anterior aspect of the spinous processes, should slope gently without sharp disruption (see Fig 8–11). Any abnormality in these lines suggests displacement. The exception is the pseudosubluxation of C-2 on C-3 due to the generalized laxity of ligaments in the infant. On the frontal projection, look for disruption of the vertebral bodies, transverse processes or pedicles, as well as paraspinal masses. The vertebral bodies are most frequently disrupted by infection or tumor, while the pedicles are disrupted by intraspinal processes. The pedicle is that portion of bone that borders the lateral aspect of the spinal cord and subarachnoid space. The medial aspects of the pedicles are convex; straightening or concavity of these pedicles denotes a lesion within the subarachnoid space or spinal cord. The transverse processes are most frequently affected by traumatic lesions.

The spinal cord and subarachnoid space are seen by CT with or without contrast material injected into the subarachnoid space. In the past, routine injection of contrast material into the subarachnoid space was followed by plain-film radiographs. However, greater resolution and ability to detect neural elements now make CT the imaging modality of choice. Specific lesions (extradural, intradural, extramedullary, and intramedullary) can be appreciated by their effect on the contrast (Fig 8–12).

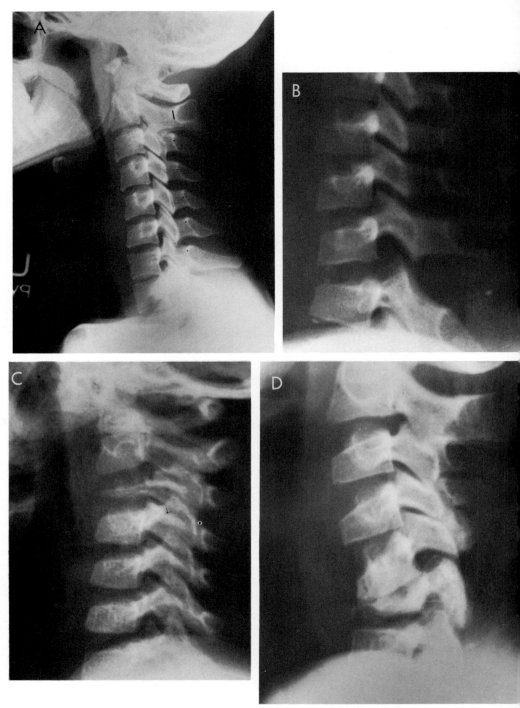

Fig 8–11.—Lateral cervical spine. **A,** normal lateral cervical spine. The dots on the vertebral process demonstrate the normal spinal curve. **B, C, D,** can you identify the abnormalities in these other childre. (See Appendix 2.)

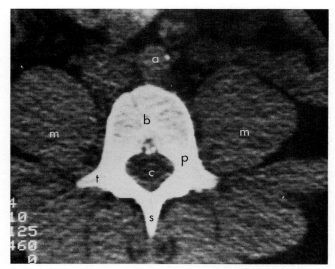

Fig 8–12.—A normal CT scan of the spine. *b,* vertebral body; *c,* spinal cord; *p,* pedicles; *t,* transverse processes; *m,* paraspinal muscles (psoas); *a,* aorta.

INDICATIONS FOR IMAGING EVALUATION

The initial evaluation remains the frontal and lateral plain film, most often supplemented by oblique views and specific odontoid films if the cervical spine is to be evaluated. The indications for this procedure include trauma, back pain (an unusual complaint in childhood), weakness of lower extremities or gait problems, unusual bladder or bowel complaints (specifically of a regressive nature), or diseases that involve metastasis to the spine. Curvature of the spine (scoliosis) and congenital anomalies of the spine (spinal dysraphism, meningomyelocele) are other indications.

A specific abnormality seen in teenagers is herniation of the nucleus pulposus—Schmorl's node—from its place in the center of the disk. This herniation may occur in any direction. When anterior, it may displace the ring epiphysis of the vertebral body, leaving the corners apparently "compressed" and the disc space narrowed (Fig 8–13). If this occurs at multiple levels, it is called Scheuermann's disease, although many children with this roentgen finding are asymptomatic.

What are the abnormalities in Figure 8–14?

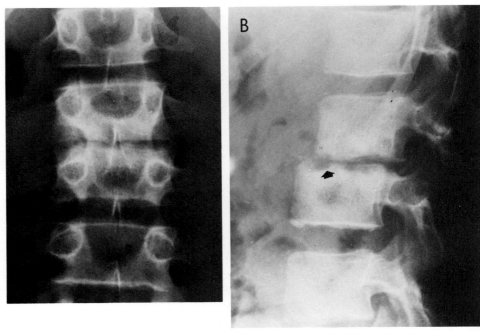

Fig 8–13.—Herniation of the nucleus pulposus—Schmorl's node. **A,** frontal view of the lumbar spine reveals narrowed disk space between L-2 and L-3 with irregular margins. **B,** lateral view shows the narrow disk space and the large AP diameter of L-3. The anterior defects *(arrows)* are sites where the nucleus pulposus has anteriorly herniated and disrupted the ring epiphysis of the vertebral body.

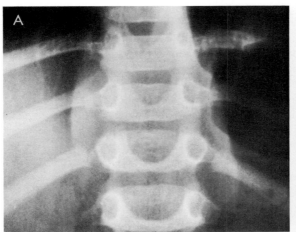

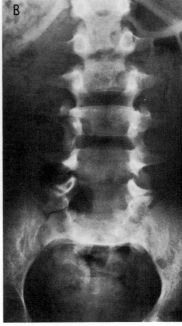

Fig 8–14.—What are these abnormalities?
(See Appendix 2.)

SUGGESTED READING

1. Harwood-Nash D.C., Hendrick E.B., Hudson A.R.: The significance of skull fracture in children—A study of 1,187 patients. *Radiology* 101:151, 1971.
2. Bell R.S., Loop J.W.: The utility and futility of radiographic skull examination for trauma. *New Engl. J. Med.* 284:236, 1971.
3. Leonidas J.C., et al.: Mild head trauma in children: When is a roentgenogram necessary? *Pediatrics* 69:132, 1982.
4. Siebert J.J., et al.: Low efficacy radiography of children. *AJR* 134:12, 1980.
5. Bell W.E., McCormick W.F.: *Increased Intracranial Pressure in Children*, ed. 2. Philadelphia, W.B. Saunders Co., 1978.
6. Shapiro R.: *Radiology of the Normal Skull.* Chicago, Year Book Medical Publishers, Inc., 1981.
7. duBoulay G.H.: *Principles of X-ray Diagnosis of the Skull*, ed. 2. London, Butterworth, 1980.
8. Keats T.E.: *Atlas of Normal Radiographic Variants*, ed. 2. Chicago, Year Book Medical Publishers, Inc., 1979.
9. Swischuk L.E.: *Radiology of the Newborn and Young Infant*, ed. 2. Baltimore, Williams & Wilkins, 1980.
10. Christenson P.D.: The Radiologic Study of the Normal Spine—Cervical, Thoracic, Lumbar and Sacral *in Radiology Clinics of North America, Symposium on the Spine*, August, 1977.

CHAPTER 9

Special Procedures

THE FIRST EIGHT chapters of this text have discussed common pediatric imaging procedures. This chapter deals with the less common, frequently more invasive procedures.

VISCERAL ANGIOGRAPHY

The last decade has seen a remarkable change in radiology. Angiography, which was the ultimate modality, has been supplanted by less invasive imaging techniques such as computerized axial tomography, sonography, and nuclear scanning. Today, in the course of a year, no more than 100 angiographic procedures would be done in a busy children's hospital; 70 of these would be cranial angiography.

The procedure is done by the percutaneous transfemoral method described in Chapter 8. Both arteries and veins can be selected in this manner, and multiple views with magnification can be obtained when indicated. Some of the more common indications for visceral angiography are listed below.

1. Renal hypertension. Allows for evaluation of the main and segmental renal arteries to detect stenosis (Fig 9–1). In addition, renal vein samplings should be obtained for renin activity.
2. Renal trauma. When surgery is anticipated, vascular supply to the remaining kidney is evaluated, allowing for a limited renal resection. Arterial-venous fistulas and false aneurysms can also be visualized.
4. Masses within the abdomen. Delineation of the vascular supply and origin of masses may be necessary when less invasive modalities are not diagnostic.
5. Hepatic masses (see Chap. 6). Angiography is important in evaluation of hepatic lesions for determining feasibility of limited resection of the liver.
6. Trauma. Evaluation of splenic rupture is certainly feasible by the angiographic technique. Usually, however, radionuclide studies provide the answer to the extent of splenic rupture. Limb trauma with vascular disruption is diagnosed by angiography.

A new modality, *digital subtraction angiography*, is a refinement of angiography. Using the digital computer system, both the arterial and venous systems can be visualized by simple injection of contrast material through a peripheral vein, obviating femoral and arterial puncture with a catheter. However, this technique is still in its infancy, and its efficacy has yet to be determined. Currently, the resolution of digital subtraction angiography is far less than that of the angiogram.

TECHNIQUES TO FURTHER EVALUATE THE AIRWAY

Magnification high-kilovoltage radiography is a noninvasive, useful procedure to delineate the upper airway, trachea, and major bronchi. The technique is most

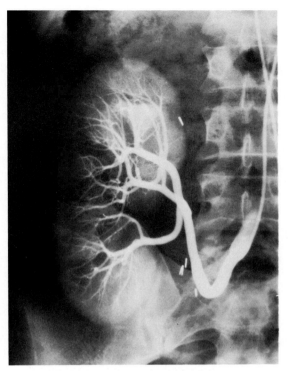

Fig 9–1.—This renal arteriogram was performed on a patient with a renal transplant (note the surgical clips) because the patient was hypertensive. This study was normal, but note the fine arterial detail seen to the periphery of the kidney.

useful for children with stridor, choking, suspected foreign body, vascular ring, and intrabronchial mass. By using a Thoreaus filter to selectively screen out low-kilovoltage radiation and by increasing the kilovoltage and magnifying the child's airway, an exquisite view is obtained. This technique has, for the most part, obviated the more invasive tracheogram, where contrast was instilled into the trachea and pictures obtained. The magnification high-KV technique can be used without sedation and with relatively little radiation.

A bronchogram may be necessary to demonstrate the more distal airway, primarily for confirmation of bronchiectasis and for demonstration of an obstructed or stenosed bronchus. For this procedure, contrast medium is injected at the carina or selectively into one bronchus. After the contrast has been injected, the patient is tilted into various positions to fill the appropriate segmental bronchi.

ARTHROGRAPHY

In older children and adolescents, the need for exquisite evaluation of the joints may arise. This is achieved by percutaneous instillation of water-soluble contrast material and air into the joint space, allowing visualization of the cartilaginous articular surfaces. Indications include suspected meniscal tears of the knees, femoral head disorders, rotator cuff tears of the shoulder, and, occasionally, ankle and foot abnormalities.

LYMPHANGIOGRAPHY

A small quantity of methylene blue is injected into the web between the first and second toes. It is rapidly taken up by lymphatic vessels, which can be seen subcutaneously passing upward on the dorsum of the foot. A small transverse incision is made over one of these lymphatics and a small portion is isolated. A fine needle is inserted into the lymphatic and injections made through a fine polyethylene catheter connecting the needle to a syringe. Iodized oil has recently been used for the injections.

Indications include evaluating the distant lymphatic nodes involved by neoplasm. It is also possible to gauge response to therapy by observing changes in the size of the lymph nodes over a period of time as shown by serial x-rays. The most common indication for this procedure is malignant disease of the lymphatic system, i.e., Hodgkin's disease.

SIALOGRAPHY

Opacification of the salivary ducts and glands by injecting contrast medium into a duct opening is usually performed to diagnose obstruction or neoplasms. The parotid gland is the one most often studied by this method.

SPLENOPORTOGRAPHY (PHLEBOGRAPHY)

This examination is performed for the investigation of portal hypertension. It is helpful in the diagnostic differentiation between intra- and extrahepatic portal obstruction. The procedure is performed by percutaneous puncture of the spleen from the flank and rapid injection of about 30 ml of concentrated intravascular contrast medium. Rapid serial films are taken over a period of some 10 seconds.

NUCLEAR MAGNETIC RESONANCE

This new technique will come to the fore in the 1980s. By placing the patient in an electromagnetic field, a computer is able to measure the spin of the various molecules in the body. Since each molecule is a dipole with a positive and negative charge, when placed in an electromagnetic field, the dipole rearranges itself. This rearrangement can be measured and translated into an image similar to that obtained by computerized axial tomography. This procedure is advantageous in that it uses no radiation.

INTERVENTIONAL RADIOGRAPHY

This new decade in radiology has seen the advent of procedures that fall under the heading of interventional radiology. They include:
1. Arterial chemotherapy infusion and arterial occlusion of malignant mass lesions
2. Arterial occlusion in arteriovenous malformations
3. Transluminal dilatation of renal artery stenosis
4. Gastrointestinal bleeding—arterial vasopressin infusion and/or embolization, as well as transhepatic variceal obliteration.

Dilatation is achieved by inserting a catheter through the stenotic lesion and blowing up a balloon so as to dilate the stenotic lesion internally. Embolization is achieved by injecting material including clot, Crazy Glue, methacrylate, coils, etc.

Under sonographic or CT guidance, biopsy samples can be obtained, using a 22-gauge Chiba needle; or antegrade studies of an obstructed or malfunctioning kidney can be performed after percutaneous puncture. Renal biopsy can be performed, and abscesses can be evacuated.

Reed's Rules

1—On every chest film, read the abdominal portion as you would read an abdominal film.
2—Knowledge of anatomy is the key to correct radiographic diagnosis.
3—The airway should be visible on all normal chest films.
4—A mass must be seen in two planes.
5—An esophagram must be done on any child with unexplained respiratory disease.
6—In unilateral hyperexpansion of the lungs, you must see how the air moves. Mediastinal position is critical to this determination.
7—Always review all old films to properly assess the new one. Subtle findings can easily be missed when a single previous examination is reviewed.
8—The abdominal examination should include a minimum of three views—supine, prone and erect.
9—On every abdominal examination, evaluate the chest as if you were looking at a chest film.
10—In obstruction of the lumen, there should be proximal distention.
11—During intravenous urography, keep taking films as long as you are getting needed information.
12—Try to find the effects of the mass on adjacent organs on each abdominal film. Draw the mass, if necessary.
13—After you have defined the mass, find the center of the lesion. Then consider all structures, gross and microscopic, near the center of the lesion as possible sources of the mass. Think skin to skin.
14—The periosteum is *not* normally seen.
15—When viewing an extremity, try to imagine the appearance of the patient. An excellent example is bowed legs or knock knees.

Answers to Questions

CHAPTER 2

Fig 2–6.—The patient in **B** is rotated to the left. The heart is appreciably in the left hemithorax, and the left side of the chest is relatively elongated, as compared to the right. The reverse is true in **A**. In **B** there are basilar densities.

Fig 2–20.—Acute epiglottitis. **A,** a 3-year-old with respiratory distress. The chest is normal, but the lateral neck shows an enlarged epiglottis and arytenoepiglottic folds.

Fig 2–38.—Unusual pulmonary densities. Frontal and lateral films of the chest reveal calcific densities beneath both hemidiaphragms. The child was asymptomatic at the time of examination. Further history revealed the patient had suffered from histoplasmosis, and these are calcified granulomas.

Fig 2–39.—A child with onset of acute respiratory distress. Did you notice the white, linear density along the right heart border? A pin was removed from the right main-stem bronchus.

Fig 2–40.—Chronic lung disease. This 13-year-old female had chronic respiratory distress of cystic fibrosis. However, there has been a sudden onset of distress. On this roentgenograph, you can see a large pneumothorax on the right side. The collapsed lung is clearly defined by extrapleural air-filled thoracic cavity. It is important to always note pleural margins of the lung. The involved lung is so diseased (stiff) that it cannot fully collapse. There is minimal shift of the mediastinum to the left.

Fig 2–41.—A child with a cough. **A,** frontal examination reveals a large density extending to the left paraspinal line behind the heart. Its borders are convex laterally *(arrows)* suggesting an extrapleural mass. **B,** on the lateral view, the mass is difficult to see. The vertebral bodies are whiter inferiorly than they are superiorly, indicating disease in the posterior aspect of the hemithorax *(arrows)*. This was a ganglioneuroblastoma.

Fig 2–42.—A child with wheezing. **A,** frontal radiograph shows the distal airway pushed to the left; the carina is not adjacent to the right pedicles. **B,** lateral film reveals the airway bowed forward and slightly narrowed *(arrows)*. **C,** frontal view of a barium swallow shows the right and left indentations on the esophagus *(arrows)*. **D,** lateral views reveal a bulge behind the esophagus *(arrow)* and some narrowing and bowing of the airway. The patient has a vascular ring, specifically a double aortic arch.

CHAPTER 3

Page 50.—Magnification of the chest occurs because of the portable technique. There is an apparent "large cardiomediastinal silhouette" because the tube-to-film distance is only 36–40 inches. Since the child is supine, the vascularity of the upper and lower lungs is equal.

CHAPTER 4

Fig 4–26.—A 9-year-old with abdominal pain. **A,** a supine film of the pelvis reveals a large mass with a calcific density in its center. **B,** ultrasonic evaluation of this patient reveals the extent of this mass *(arrows).* A teratoma was removed. *b,* bladder; *h,* cephalad; *a,* anterior; *f,* caudad; *u,* uterus.

Fig 4–27.—An infant with abdominal distention. A supine film reveals air-filled bowel within the inguinal canals. These are bilateral inguinal hernias *(arrows).*

Fig 4–28.—Abdominal pain after trauma. A plain film of the abdomen is unremarkable. Contrast was given by mouth, and there was an abrupt change in the size and contour of the duodenum in its horizontal portion. The wall is effaced, that is, the mucosal pattern is stretched over a submucosal mass, which is a duodenal hematoma.

Fig 4–29.—Two neonates with abdominal distention. **A,** there is extraluminal gas in the descending colon (linear black streaks) *(arrow).* This is pneumatosis intestinalis or air in the wall of the bowel. **B,** another infant with necrotizing enterocolitis has portal venous gas *(arrow).* There is abdominal distention, but the pneumatosis is not as clearly defined.

CHAPTER 5

Fig 5–5.—What abnormalities do you see? **A,** an infant who had the bladder filled during a VCU. A portion of the bladder wall has herniated into the inguinal canal *(arrow).* These are called "bladder ears" and are of no clinical significance. **B,** an IVU in a 7 ½-year-old who was in an automobile accident. The upper tracts appear normal, but the bladder is raised off the pelvic floor. There is obvious disruption of the left pubic bone. **C,** same patient as **B.** A retrograde study was performed, and the catheter was removed. There is contrast in the pelvis because of disruption of the posterior urethra. Contrast in the left hip joint indicates disruption of the bones of the acetabulum as well.

Fig 5–7.—Multiple abnormal IVUs. **A,** a 10-year-old with a left flank mass. This is a 10 minute film. The right kidney appears normal, but on the left, there is a large mass with linear densities *(arrows).* The densities represent the parenchymal tubules being pushed in a vertical direction (parenchymal rims about a more lucent, dilated urine-filled collecting system). **B,** a coned-down view of this kidney shows the rims to better advantage. This patient had ureteropelvic junction obstruction. **C,** a 5-minute film from a 6-year-old with repeated urinary tract infections. The left kidney *(arrow)* is considerably smaller than the right and measures less than 3 vertebral bodies in height. The right kidney is larger than normal, measuring just about 5 vertebral bodies in height. **D,** an 8-year-old with urinary tract infection and high fever. The upper-pole calix of the right kidney *(arrow)* is farther from the spine than one would expect (see left upper-pole calix *[arrow]*). A palpable mass in this clinical setting is most consistent for a renal abscess.

Fig 5–10.—Multiple abnormalities detected on ultrasound. **A,** longitudinal, supine scan showing an anechoic region *(arrows)* with good sound transmission and posterior enhancement at the upper pole of the right kidney *(k).* **B,** urogram on the same child shows lateral displacement of the calices in the right upper pole. This child had a simple renal cyst. **C,** prone, longitudinal scan in an 8-year-old with urinary tract infection reveals dilatation of the lower-pole central collecting system.

The central sinus echoes are separated *(arrows)*, with the upper pole being normal. **D,** urogram demonstrates a double left collecting system with dilatation of the lower pole on the basis of reflux. **E,** a 15-year-old with a neurogenic bladder. This longitudinal, supine scan of the right kidney shows separation of the central sinus echoes (see normal scan, Fig 5–9,*C*). *L* = liver. **F,** urogram at the same time shows bilateral hydronephrosis and hydroureter (the latter also seen by ultrasound examination).

CHAPTER 7

Fig 7–11.—The lateral epicondyle is displaced inferiorly due to a fracture through the apophyseal growth plate. Sometimes subtle growth-plate injuries require comparison views of the other extremity.

Fig 7–13.—There are posterior rib fractures of the left fifth, sixth, seventh, and eighth ribs.

Fig 7–24.—**A,** benign bone cyst of the calcaneus. It is a solitary lesion which has a clear zone of demarcation, no periosteal reaction, and a single lucency, typical of a cyst. You certainly thought this was benign, didn't you? **B,** Legg-Calvé-Perthes disease, or aseptic necrosis. The child complained of left hip pain, and the left femoral head appears somewhat shallower and flatter than the right. Note the defect at the most lateral aspect of the growth plate. These findings are typical of early aseptic necrosis. **C,** film of patient in **B,** taken 6 months later, showing the sequela of this disease. There is fragmentation of the femoral head and broadening of the femoral neck. The appendicolith that was present on the previous film (did you spot it?) was removed when the patient presented a month before admission with appendicitis. **D,** Brodie's abscess. The sclerosis at the posterior aspect of the proximal tibia diaphysis is a clue. A lucency can be seen in the center, and the differential diagnoses include infections such as a Brodie's abscess, osteoid osteoma, and healing fracture.

CHAPTER 8

Fig 8–10.—Compare the pedicles. The left pedicle of L-5 is dense when compared to the right pedicle or to either pedicle of L-4. This is a common location for an osteoid osteoma, which is a benign bone lesion causing pain.

Fig 8–11.—**B,** Careful attention to the vertical lines reveals that C-7, the lowest cervical vertebra, is out of position. Look at the relationship of the articulating facets. This is a dislocation of C-7.

Fig 8–11.—**C,** are all the vertebral bodies the same height? C-2 is a "wafer" vertebra. The joint space is intact, but the vertebral body is severely compressed. This is commonly found in eosinophilic granuloma of bone.

Fig 8–11.—**D,** a compression fracture of C-4. Trauma is a major cause of vertebral compression fractures and wedging.

Fig. 8–14.—**A,** tuberculosis; Pott's disease. Note the disk space narrowing of T11-12. The bilateral paraspinal masses may calcify as they heal. **B,** meningomyelocele. You should have detected the bifid spinous processes of L-2 and the absent posterior elements of L-3 through L-5. Did you note that the pedicles have lost their convex inner margins, suggesting an interspinal mass? This is a meningomyelocele with open posterior elements.

Index